The Arthritis Diet Cookbook

MICHAEL MCILWRAITH is a fellow of the Hotel Catering & Institutional Management Association, and is widely known to professional colleagues as a pioneer of modern methods of hospital catering. Trained as a chef, he has also worked in Hotel Management but is now retired and devotes his time to writing about food and to travelling with his wife, Mollie Hunter. They live in the Highlands of Scotland.

MOLLIE HUNTER is an award-winning writer of books for children and young adults and her work has been translated into many languages.

The Arthritis Diet Cookbook

MICHAEL McILWRAITH FHCIMA

Foreword by Mollie Hunter

LONDON
VICTOR GOLLANCZ LTD
1988

First published in Great Britain May 1988
by Victor Gollancz Ltd,
14 Henrietta Street, London WC2E 8QJ
Second impression May 1988

First published in Gollancz Paperbacks 1988

British Library Cataloguing in Publication Data
McIlwraith, Michael
    The arthritis diet cookbook: how one
    woman helped herself to fitness.
    1. Arthritis—Diet therapy—Recipes
    I. Title
    616.7'220654   RC933

    ISBN 0-575-04288-5
    ISBN 0-575-04265-6 Pbk

Phototypeset by Rowland Phototypesetting Ltd,
Bury St Edmunds, Suffolk
Printed in Finland by Werner Söderström Oy

To Herself,
mistress of my heart and of my home

Contents

Foreword

I have rheumatoid arthritis – a condition I share with more than a million people in Great Britain. The fact of your having this book now in your hands points therefore to one of two possibilities. Either you too have the disease, or – with such a high incidence of its occurrence being the case – you know someone who suffers from it.

That person may be one who is affected in only a few of their joints, or who may experience to only a minimal degree the characteristic joint inflammation and subsequent pain. On the other hand, it could as easily be one who has numerous joints affected, for whom the inflammation is acute, the pain so severe as to be indescribable, and the resultant disablement almost total. I write with feeling of these more unfortunate ones, since I have been numbered among them.

Have been? No cure has been found as yet for rheumatoid arthritis. Nor does anything that follows here purport to be a cure. All of which being so, how can I admit to still having the disease at the same time as stating myself to be once again mobile in all my joints and free now of the pain I once suffered? The answer to that question, I believe, lies in the fact that I follow the diet which is later described in this book; and so, for the benefit of others who might also contemplate taking up that same diet, a brief account of the circumstances that led me to do so would appear to be in order.

The disease first struck me in the middle of my sixty-second year when my hands suddenly became grossly swollen and extremely painful. Since I am a writer by profession it can be imagined how much I was dismayed then to find myself physically incapable of using a typewriter or even of holding a pen in my hand; nor did the anti-inflammatory drug that was prescribed do anything to decrease the swelling or to ease the pain of trying to use those tools of my trade.

A few months after this first onset of the disease, however, my husband and I had the good fortune to spend several weeks with friends in Florida; and by the end of the first week there the pain and swelling in my hands had become rather less. This improvement continued to be the case, and on our return home I was told that I had probably experienced a natural remission of my illness. This, I was also told, is something that quite commonly happens to those struck in the way that had happened with me – as, indeed, I later learned, can frequently also be the case with any victim of rheumatoid arthritis.

The situation as it was with me then continued to be so for another few months, during which time we in this country were blessed with very warm weather – a fact which seemed to strengthen our supposition that the warm weather first experienced in Florida could have played at least a part in bringing about and then continuing this happy state of affairs.

Then came the blow of the disease returning to afflict me in severe and widespread form. Except for the hips and spine, all my joints were this time affected by it, and there was neither improvement nor relief to be had from any of the half-dozen or so anti-inflammatory drugs that were tried against it. A different type of drug was therefore prescribed; but as this was one that can have severe side-effects, the dosage was kept at sub-therapeutic level until it could be determined whether or not my system could tolerate it. The further treatment recommended involved a spell in hospital, and to this I agreed – as I would have agreed then to anything, however drastic, that held out for me any hope of minimising the pain.

Going into hospital was a shattering experience. For the first time in my life I was brought into close daily contact with people who had been dreadfully crippled by rheumatoid arthritis. I could see my own future mirrored in their condition, and the depression that took hold of me then was extreme. I was not alone in this, however, since – as I very quickly learned – depression can very often be a feature of this illness, and the patients were as mutually supportive in this respect as they were with one another in all other aspects of their various conditions.

The hospital course lasted for six weeks, and consisted of a regime that carefully integrated periods of rest and relaxation with painkilling drugs and other periods of intensive physiotherapy. I emerged from the course vastly improved in every way. Also, since it had been established by then that, despite some

distinctly unpleasant side-effects, my system could tolerate the
drug I had been prescribed shortly before entering hospital, the
dosage of this was increased to what was presumed to be a
therapeutic level.

A further holiday in a warm climate was what then seemed
advisable, the supposition my husband and I had formed of the
benefits of Florida sunshine still being very much alive with us. In
high hope therefore that the combination of the prescribed drug,
sunny weather, and persistence with the physical exercises I had
been taught in hospital would sustain my improved condition, we
took off again – this time, to Spain.

For the month that this holiday lasted, my improvement also
lasted. After this, however, my condition began steadily to de-
teriorate again until I was first of all no longer capable of doing my
daily exercises and was finally reduced to an even worse state than
had been the case before entering hospital. I was, in fact, in
constant pain, as well as being immobilised to the point of being
almost completely unable to perform the smallest action. United
opinion was that I had no option except to go back into hospital –
united, that is, except for my own feelings on the subject.

All my life until the disease struck me I had been physically very
active, and I was determined that what remained of that life was
not going to be spent in repeating spells of hospitalisation. The
drug prescribed for me had apparently been powerless to prevent
the relapse to my then low state; and I was equally determined
that the rest of my life was not going to be spent in the type of vain
search I had seen others following in pursuit of some drug that
would be effective against the disease. By that time also, I had read
everything I could find on the subject of rheumatoid arthritis, and
had at least been able to establish certain facts about it.

The cause of the disease is still unknown. On that, all medical
opinion is agreed. The onset is indicated by one or more joints of
the body becoming inflamed; and once this happens, the body's
tissues and defence mechanisms give the impression of reacting
against themselves and so perpetuating the inflammatory process.
There is no apparent reason for the initial inflammatory process;
but it would also seem to be generally held opinion that there is
some sort of "trigger factor" behind it. The logical assumption
from the foregoing is that, if the trigger factor could be identified,
some way could be found of dealing with its effects, and there is

today much experimentation going on towards that end – which is heartening.

Much of this experimentation, also, has focused on the question of diet, particularly those foods which have high levels of animal fat and consumption of which leads in turn to high levels of cholesterol in the blood. Patients with rheumatoid arthritis have been found to benefit from reduction of their intake of this animal or "saturated" fat and replacement of it with polyunsaturates; and the postulate from this has been that the body's development of allergy towards saturated fat could be the trigger factor.

It has been noted also that among those peoples (Japanese, Eskimos) who have a high fish intake in their diet, there is a low incidence of rheumatoid arthritis; and this has been connected with the fact that fish oils are rich in eicosapentaenoic acid, a substance which is known to restrict the way in which the body responds to inflammation. To combine a diet of foods avoiding animal fats with a daily intake of fish oil capsules seemed thus to offer a hopeful line of experiment; and this, when tried recently in the USA, did indeed have a high rate of success in reducing the symptoms of patients with rheumatoid arthritis.

It was after reading of the American experiment that I reached the low point where I had been told I must go back into hospital, and so I was then in the classic situation of having everything to gain and nothing to lose by attempting to proceed on the lines it had followed. My husband had also read of the experiment. Indeed, since his profession is food, he had read far more deeply than I would ever be able to do on the whole question of therapeutic diet. He was in complete agreement with my decision that I should give the diet theory a chance to work in my case; and, he assured me, the one I proposed to follow would not only answer completely to all modern concepts of healthy eating, it was also one that could be made both varied and appetising. That would simply be a matter of selectivity in the first instance, and then of modifying recipes to widen the range of choice available.

To ensure, then, that the diet was given a really fair trial, I began methodically on my change of eating habits and continued to be as methodical in recording the results. First of all, I informed my doctor of my intentions – something it is generally advisable to do before starting any kind of diet, but which becomes an essential step in any situation where one is receiving medication from the doctor.

I bought a supply of the fish oil capsules which were used in the American experiment and which are marketed in this country under the brand name of "Maxepa" and which now, incidentally, are also available on prescription from any sympathetic GP. Then, to clear out my system, as it were, I had Day 1 entirely without food, but was careful to drink plenty of water. On Day 2, I had nothing except raw vegetables and water, after which I was ready to eat all that could properly be considered part of the diet.

From the very beginning, also, I followed a practice which I thought then and still think is essential to anyone in my situation. I kept a daily record of every item eaten and drunk, together with a detailed account of symptoms experienced, and any treatment given to affected joints in terms either of heat from an infra-red lamp, or of ice-packs. Exercise was something that could not be recorded at first in my diary, since I then had only minimal use of my joints. My husband, however, was very willing to take me to the local swimming baths. There, immersed up to my neck and with the buoyancy of the water to aid me, I was able to perform various gentle movements; and with a record kept also of this form of exercise, I then had the complete information needed to assess my progress.

The first full day of the diet for me was 10th June 1985. Throughout the following ten days I experienced various small hopeful signs; but even so, by the time 20th June arrived, I was still at the lowest point I had ever reached. From this time on, I began to show sporadic signs of improvement, gaining ground one day, losing some of this the next, but still improving overall. By 1st July I was able to record my first night's sleep without pain since beginning the diary; by 4th July, the fact that I had been able to extend my exercises in the baths until I was actually swimming; and by 5th July, to record that I had experienced my best day since starting the diary.

The further improvement that followed was achieved at a steady rate. The swelling in my hands decreased until they looked almost normal. The pain in various joints became less and less, and the mobility of all joints was increased. I extended my range of activities to walking, and a little gentle gardening. At the baths, I reached the point where I could dive in from the side and swim freely. By 20th July I was able to ride a bicycle, and did so to pay a visit to my doctor who was both amazed and delighted to see me thus arriving at his surgery.

"Something", he pronounced, "has done you a lot of good – and it's nothing *I've* given you." Upon which he cut the dosage of my prescribed drug in half and made an appointment for me to see the Consultant Rheumatologist. When the time came for my appointment, the Consultant expressed his views in precisely the words my doctor had used.

"Something", he pronounced, "has done you a lot of good – and it's nothing *I've* given you." Whereupon he cut out the drug altogether.

This was on 29th July, seven weeks after starting the diet. In the middle of August I spent a week at the Edinburgh Festival Book Fair where my latest novel was being launched amid scenes of considerable publicity. All my friends in the book trade remarked then on how well I looked, and I still have the photographs of these scenes to prove the truth of their remarks. It was during this time of celebration, also, that two things happened with regard to my diet.

I ventured on white wine which, along with all other forms of alcohol, had been banished from my diet simply on the general principle that alcohol isn't good for one in any case. There was no adverse reaction from the wine, and I have since gone back to my usual moderate habits in that respect. There was, however, one definitely adverse reaction from a dish (duck) which is forbidden in the diet, and I spent an extremely unpleasant few hours in a radio station wrestling with a return of arthritic pain instead of being able to concentrate on the programme in which I was taking part.

Back home again, I settled into the routine I had always followed previous to having the disease, and which I was now once more happily able to observe. But with one difference, of course – this being the application of the lesson I had learned in hospital on the importance of daily exercising all my joints and muscles. Additionally, I continued with my thrice-weekly swimming sessions, this being a form of exercise I found highly enjoyable as well as one that served the very practical purpose of strengthening muscles debilitated by the fact of my having for so long been unable to use them.

To give my final assessment then, some three years after starting my diet and having stuck faithfully to it during all that time, I can now truthfully say that I am as well as I was before the disease struck me. I have occasional reminders, of course, that it is still with me – a twinge of pain now and then, or sometimes before I settle for sleep a tingling in my legs or the soles of my feet. But even these slight phenomena, I hope, will pass in the course of time; and even if they do not, what are they compared to the ferocious pain and the disability I have had previously to suffer?

I still also experience a certain occasional stiffness in my joints and do not have the power in these that I once had. But I am, after all, sixty-five years old. I can, and do, walk briskly for several hours at a time, ride a bicycle, and swim three times a week. And so, how much more active would a person of my age normally be? As for other forms of activity, I spend approximately six hours a day at my writing work; and that work also involves me in frequent speaking engagements which, in themselves, further involve me in extensive travelling both in this country and in others far afield of it.

When at home, also, I share with my husband the running of an eight-roomed house, the tending of a very large garden, and the occasional care of our three grandsons: all of which inclines me occasionally to be thankful that I have continued to observe the other lesson I learned in hospital – namely, that regular rest of all the joints and muscles affected by rheumatoid arthritis is as vital in maintaining their wellbeing as is regular exercise.

As for that sunny weather which my husband and I once thought could have been a chief factor in lessening the symptoms of rheumatoid arthritis, it is undoubtedly the case that pain creates tension in joints and muscles; and that warmth, by helping one to relax the tension must inevitably therefore play a part in reducing the pain.

Nevertheless, having weathered the very worst that the climate of northern Scotland could produce during the extremely wet summer and the extremely cold winter we experienced here in my first nine months on the diet, it would seem that the really important thing in this respect is simply to wear the kind of clothing that will keep the joints warm, and thus help also to keep them supple.

There is still one important point missing, however, from all the observations I have so far made on the change that the diet has brought to my circumstances. I have said that I have followed it faithfully from that very first day on 10th June 1985. But has this been hard to do? Don't I miss the kind of food I used to eat? Do I really *enjoy* the diet? The answer to all these questions is, quite simply, that I have never eaten better in my life – and I am a person who likes my food to the point where, at my age at least, I have to watch my weight. But on this diet (unless, of course, one is greedy) one does not put on weight – as happens all too often, unfortunately, with even moderate indulgence of the foods that are forbidden in it.

Finally then, to the question that must be in the minds of all who have read to this point. Is it really the diet that has made such a difference to me, or has it simply been that I have experienced a natural remission of my rheumatoid arthritis coincidentally with beginning to live according to the diet? This is a question I myself wanted to have answered, and so I put it to my own doctor.

He offered no opinion on the diet as such, except to agree that it was certainly one conducive to good health; but on the subject of remission his opinion was that the general nature of the change in my condition did not bear out what had previously been his experience of what was usually taken to be a natural remission. One other point on which we were agreed was that, although research so far has been insufficient to produce hard scientific evidence one way or another, there is certainly enough empirical evidence to justify a doctor supporting a patient who wishes to experiment with diet as a means of combatting rheumatoid arthritis. And in my own experience of late, there are more and more doctors who are doing so.

The obvious corollary to the foregoing, of course, is co-operation with one's doctor, first in discussing with him/her the intention to go on the diet, and second with continuing such medication as may have been prescribed until – as happened with me – one's medical advisers decide that the condition achieved means that there is no longer any point to continuing with it.

Having brought you this far, then, the rest is up to you. Would you rather live with pain and drugs (some of which have proved to be very harmful)? Would you rather have someone dear to you live in such a way? Or would you rather give the diet a try? That question has long been answered for me; but even so, my memories of what life used to be like for me are so vivid that I still greet each active and pain-free new day like a person reborn. And so, if you do decide to follow my example in this, *Bon appétit* – and the very best of my good wishes for *your* future.

Mollie Hunter

Introduction to the Diet

This book has been inspired by my work in adapting recipes to suit Mollie's diet.

There were no problems for me, of course, in the actual process of adaptation. As a hospital catering manager with over thirty years' experience of food preparation in all types of hospitals, I was able to draw on extensive practical knowledge of adapting recipes to suit not only therapeutic diets, but also a great variety of tastes and prejudices. Yet even so, there was a considerable degree of research and experiment required in order to evolve the range of dishes needed to give reasonable variation over an extended span of time.

The diet to be followed called for *elimination of all animal fats*; and yet, animal fats are contained in all dairy products, yolk of egg, and in red meats such as beef, mutton and pork where (although this is not apparently so) it occurs even in the muscle. Most recipes, also, call for the use of butter and egg, milk and cream. All made-up meat dishes contain animal fat in some degree. Sausages, pies, pâtés, hamburgers, and all sorts of convenience foods from tins and deep-freeze were therefore also taboo.

Indications from both sides of the Atlantic, nevertheless, were that diet *could* help those suffering from rheumatoid arthritis; and there was general agreement about animal fats. There was some controversy as to which other foods could be tolerated and which could not. Most opinion seemed to be against cereals. Some schools of thought banned most fruits and even some vegetables. So far as the controversial items were concerned, however, I was fortunate inasmuch that recent experience had offered some guidance.

Mollie and I had just returned from a holiday in Spain where we had gone in the belief that sun and low humidity would continue the beneficial effect of her stay in hospital. Something did indeed do so, and no doubt the sun was a contributory factor; but when we came seriously to consider diet and looked back on this

Spanish interlude, we remembered also what we had eaten in the course of it.

We had taken a self-catering apartment, so that we were in complete control of our menu; and because we believe in "doing in Rome as the Romans do", we followed the Spanish practice of cooking in olive oil, rather than in butter. We ate very little red meat, preferring fish (of which a great deal is eaten in Spain), also poultry, and the plentiful fresh salads that were available. Because we liked the Spanish *barra* (a long loaf similar to the French *baguette*) we ate a great deal of this kind of bread; and when it came to fruit, we found we could not resist the large, sweet Valencia oranges, of which we devoured huge quantities.

Looking back on our other experience in the sun after the disease first attacked Mollie, we further remembered our diet while we were in Florida. There again, as in Spain, we indulged ourselves in the luscious oranges surrounding us. We took full advantage of the super salad bars which are a feature of all American restaurants. Because of the food preferences of our hosts we ate very little meat, but, reflecting the enormous range of fish available, we ate fish oftener than we normally would have done. We avoided the Americans' dreadful additive-laden store bread; but whenever we could get it we ate what they call "ethnic bread" – e.g. French bread, Italian bread, bagels, and English muffins.

Our conclusions from all this were that, as Mollie's condition had improved during both the Spain and the Florida interlude, it was most unlikely that the consumption of fruit and cereals was an adverse factor in her condition. Nevertheless, since other commentators had made much of the suggestion that rheumatoid arthritis sufferers cannot tolerate the high acid content of fruit, and in view also of a widely-recognised incidence of allergy to cereals – particularly wheat – I erred at first on the side of caution in including these items in the diet. My advice to arthritis sufferers in general is to follow this same practice.

Let's get back now to that word "diet". To most people it is one that implies restrictions of all kinds on indulging in the food they most enjoy. For anyone contemplating this particular diet, cutting out steaks and chops, butter, cream, cheese – and even the humble boiled egg! – the future might at first glance appear to be a bleak one. But this, fortunately, is very far from being the case. There is still an enormously wide range of foods available, all of them suitable for the arthritis diet, all of them either attractive to the palate or capable of being prepared in ways to make them so.

Far from limiting one's choice, in fact, this diet actually frees it from many restrictions imposed simply by habit and custom. It is all a matter of having the necessary recipes available in a form that the ordinary household cook can easily follow; and that is the aim of this book. There has been no attempt at *cordon bleu* cookery, no searching for new way-out recipes. All effort has been directed to adapting recipes for everyday usage. It is true, of course, that reference has been made here and there to such exotic items as Beluga caviar and pâté de foie gras Strasbourg, but this is simply because there will always be occasions such as the twenty-first birthday party or the golden wedding celebration, and it will be useful then to know which of these seldom-encountered dishes are suitable for the diet.

A further aim of this book is to provide recipes which will appeal to the whole family and not only to the arthritis sufferer. This is an extremely important aspect of coping with diet, since most people would like to be seen to be living as normal a life as possible, rather than seeming to be singled out in some way. On a practical level, it causes less work for the cook if special dishes do not have to be individually prepared. It is tedious, after all, to have to make up one portion of a particular dish; and the further aspect of this is that it encourages the easy option of providing only fast-food dishes for the diet. This, of course – as well as being limiting – can also be wasteful!

Although my primary purpose in writing this book is to help those afflicted by rheumatoid arthritis, it is my belief that these low cholesterol recipes can also help people who are suffering from heart disease, or who are potential sufferers.

This last-mentioned group is very large and growing all the time, because the present diet of the great mass of people in the Western world brings them all under threat. Small groups of doctors from all over Europe and America have been for years sounding the alarm on this. Now the medical profession in general is telling us loudly and clearly that bad eating habits are a main contributing factor in heart disease; and a chief culprit in this has proved to be animal fats. The diet outlined in this book completely avoids the use of animal fats, and will therefore be highly beneficial also to those suffering from or threatened by heart disease.

Another factor to be considered is that, if one is afflicted either by heart disease or arthritis it makes sense not to be overweight; and, since many items such as milk and cream, bacon fat and suet are excluded from this diet to be replaced only partially by others such as oil and lean meat, there will probably be an initial weight loss for anyone starting on it. But take care. While the recipes in the book are designed to be enjoyed, too much enjoyment will expand the waistline. Nor is there any way to avoid that fact. The magic pill that reduces weight simply does not exist.

Weight-reducing diets there are by the hundreds, of course; but there is only one certain as well as safe way to lose weight. That is, to eat less. The diet that works is a diet that controls intake.

With some people, however, the situation is that their bodies are more efficient at converting food into stored fat than is the case with others. To put that situation at its extreme, one person appears to be able to stay slim on a diet of suet pudding and chocolate, while another seems to gain weight on nothing more than small portions of salad.

It still applies, nevertheless, that however little the overweight may feel they are eating, they should and must *eat less right across the whole range of food*. To eat nothing but grapefruit for a week can be dangerous. We all need a varied diet that includes protein, carbohydrate, fats, and the vitamins and minerals that occur in fresh fruits and vegetables. But don't get into the mathematics of calories, kilocalories, and joules. It's all too complicated. Sufficient to know that the real heavyweights in the calorie brigade are the fats.

Olive oil contains five times as many calories as lean meat, and margarine four times as many. Both add weight as efficiently as butter or lard; and changing to polyunsaturated fat therefore does nothing to reduce weight. What must be borne in mind is that extra weight is gained over a period, and it should be lost over a period. To achieve this, you must eat just a little less at each meal. Cut the bread for the morning toast a little thinner, and go easy on the marmalade. You will, in any case, be cutting out biscuits from "elevenses", because biscuits contain butter; but don't replace them with tuna-fish sandwiches. Do not load the vegetables with melted margarine – and resist the temptation of that last potato in the dish!

I must briefly make reference here also to the subject of *additives*. While the diet outlined in this book excludes packaged convenience foods (and therefore many of those additives generally considered injurious to health), there is still a wide range of foodstuffs that may contain additives which it would be advisable to avoid. There are many excellent books on this subject, and I advise consulting one of these.

I hope that success with the recipes in this book will encourage you to look further afield for other dishes which will be suitable for the diet. A look through the recipes from countries other than our own could be profitable. They can all offer something which will widen your choice; but most will require adapting. For example, many traditional dishes from eastern Europe and Scandinavia include sour cream. Recipes from the Balkans and the Middle East add yoghurt, India swims in *ghee*, and Italy seems to add cheese to everything. All, however, have dishes which use none of these forbidden foods, and many of the recipes are well worth adapting.

It is the vegetarians, strangely enough, who have perhaps the least to offer. They eat no fish or poultry, but they do use a great deal of dairy produce. On the credit side, however, what they can contribute are many novel ways of preparing cereals, pulses, and pastas, all of which provide dishes that are very interesting and most suitable for the diet.

Finally, the probability is that (as happens with weight increase) the situation causing harm to your body was one that built up gradually, and that your reaction to the harmful agent(s) will therefore reduce gradually. And so, persevere! With some people improvement appears after about three weeks. With others, it takes longer. You can afford to take the time it requires for you – there are no side-effects! I know from personal experience that this diet has helped many people, and my hope is that it will help many more.

Soya Products

Soya Milk

Soya milk, which must be used as a substitute for dairy milk in this diet, can be bought in cartons, or in concentrated form in tins, from any health food shop. It is quite easy to make, however, and it is considerably cheaper to do so.

To prepare, soak 1 cupful of soya beans for at least 10 hrs. Thoroughly wash the beans, and divide into three portions. Using a liquidiser, blend each portion with ½ pint of boiling water. (If you have a large enough food processor you may be able to blend all the beans in one operation.) Pour the total quantity of blended beans into a jelly bag or fine muslin strainer.

Using a wooden spoon, squeeze out as much milk as possible. Pour a further pint of boiling water through the mixture in the jelly bag, and again squeeze it as dry as possible. Pour the milk into a large pan – at least 6-pint size, as the milk boils over very easily. Simmer for 5–6 mins, stirring constantly to prevent burning. Cool quickly. Store in fridge in clean bottles. It will keep for 3–4 days.

Bean Curd

There are two types of bean curd, both of which can make valuable contributions to this diet. The tougher version – which is the one that Chinese restaurants serve fried – is as yet, unfortunately, available only in Chinese provision shops. It *can* be prepared in the home, but this is a task for the enthusiast. *Tofu* is the other of the two types of bean curd. It is of Japanese origin, and is sold in cartons in all health food shops as "Silken Tofu". I have made only brief reference in this book to tofu, but it has a wide range of usage and details of this can be found in pamphlets and books which are readily available in health food stores.

TVP (Textured Vegetable Protein)

This is a processed soya bean extract which, when reconstituted by soaking in water, has the texture and the appearance of meat. In itself, it is quite tasteless, and so must take its flavour from the ingredients of the dish to which it has been added. A "meat flavoured" version is available, but because of the additives this contains, it is not recommended. Full details of its various uses are again available in health food stores.

Alcohol

I have frequently been asked what effect alcohol may have on those following this diet, and the simple answer is: "I do not know."

Different writers on this subject, after all, have given such widely varying opinions, that there would appear to be no really clear-cut answer. I can safely state, however, from my own personal observation of a number of cases of people following this diet, that a moderate amount of alcohol does not appear to have any ill-effects.

My advice, therefore, is that you should play safe by cutting out all consumption of alcohol until you are established on the diet and can assess its effects on you. You may then reasonably introduce the occasional glass of white wine. Red wine, and spirits of any kind, should definitely be avoided at this stage. Take care to note whether or not your occasional glass of white wine creates any adverse reaction. If it does, then it is fairly obvious that you cannot tolerate alcohol. But even if it does not and you therefore feel safe to increase your consumption, you should still bear in mind that alcohol is a drug, to be treated cautiously, and used with restraint.

Stocks

We depend on good stock to impart flavour to so many dishes that it is worth while always to have some available. A home-made stock offers no problems for this diet, provided all fat is removed. Avoid the temptation to use a stock cube because it is easier. Stock cubes contain a high percentage of animal fat and a number of undesirable additives. Furthermore, the artificial flavour enhancers used in stock cubes impart a sameness of taste which permeates everything, swamping more delicate flavours.

Chicken Stock
Makes 1 qt

> chicken giblets
> neck
> carcass, raw or cooked
> 1 onion
> 1 bay leaf
> 2 pt water

Simmer the chicken remains with the onion and bay leaf for 1 hr. Strain and cool. When quite cold, any fat can easily be lifted off. This is much easier to do than skimming fat from hot stock.

White Vegetable Stock
Makes 1 qt

> 1 onion, roughly chopped
> 1 carrot
> 1 turnip
> tops of few celery sticks
> 1 Tbsp vegetable oil *or* margarine
> 2 pt water
> green of leek
> 1 bay leaf
> *Optional* trimmings of cabbage, cauliflower,
>   parsnips, potato

Sweat the onion, carrot, and turnip in the oil. Add the water.

Throw in the celery and leeks (and other trimmings, as desired) and simmer for 1 hr.

Other trimmings should be well washed beforehand. Strain and use same day if possible. The stock *may* be kept in a refrigerator overnight, but vegetable stock quickly goes off.

Brown Vegetable Stock

Follow same method as for White Vegetable Stock, except that the onion should not be peeled. Cut the onion in half and place directly on to a red-hot plate, and burn it completely black. With gas – hold it on a long fork over a low flame until burned black. Place the onion pieces, whole, into the stock, and boil without breaking up the onion. This is the method used in French kitchens to colour consommé to a golden-brown.

Fish Stock

The best fish stock is considered to be made from flat fish. Beg bones and heads from your fishmonger. Cover them well with cold water. Add a roughly-chopped onion, 1 bay leaf, and a few peppercorns. Bring slowly to the boil, and simmer for 30 mins. Strain through a cloth.

Roux and Beurre Manié

These thickening agents have the same ingredients, but are mixed in different quantities and are used at different stages of the cooking process.

Roux

This is a mixture of equal quantities of fat and flour. The fat is melted and the flour stirred in. For a white roux, it is cooked a little, but not allowed to brown. The stock is then added gradually. This is used when a sauce is prepared separately or at the beginning of a cooking process, and it is then cooked with the dish. A brown roux is prepared by cooking the flour and fat mixture to a nut-brown colour – be careful not to burn. It is used for brown sauces and stews.

When making a roux for thickening soups or sauces, plain or wholemeal flour is usually used but I find that self-raising flour is most useful for this purpose. The raising agent helps it to break down more easily, and so helps to avoid lumps. The taste of the baking powder does not come through in the most delicate of sauces but self-raising flour makes the roux so much easier to mix into the soup or sauce or whatever.

Beurre Manié

This is prepared with a little less flour than fat (we use margarine) – about 75% of the weight of the fat. Mix the flour and fat to a paste, and shake, rather than stir, into a cooked dish. Bring the dish to simmering, but do not allow to boil. If it boils, it will taste floury, and have to be cooked further.

Court Bouillon   *Per qt of water*

    1 bay leaf
    1 bouquet garni
    salt
    a few peppercorns
    2 Tbsp vinegar

Add all the ingredients to the water.

Court Bouillon is not a stock, but is the traditional cooking liquor for large fish. The more conservative cooks still use it but the modern tendency is just to use salted water.

Bouquet Garni

Used to impart herb flavours to stock. A genuine bouquet garni is prepared by wrapping sprigs of fresh herbs in the green of leek, or celery, then tying them in a bundle; and this is still the best method. If you do not have access to fresh herbs, the alternative is to tie some dried herbs into a piece of muslin. In either case, leave a foot or so of the tying string free, and attach this to the handle of the pot, so that the bouquet can be easily removed. You can also find packets of ready-made bouquet garni in any food market. The most popular combination of herbs is parsley, thyme, and bay leaf, but any preferred combination of aromatic herbs can be used.

Sauces

This section is probably the most important part of the book. A sauce is what turns boiled sole into Sole Véronique, or grilled steak into Steak Béarnaise. Unfortunately, the traditional methods of preparing nearly all sauces rule them out absolutely from the diet. It is possible, however, to prepare most acceptable substitutes, some of which would require a very discerning palate indeed to distinguish them from the traditional recipe.

White Sauce (Béchamel) *Makes ½ pt*

    1 oz margarine
    1 oz flour
    ¼ pt stock
    ¼ pt soya milk
    1 small onion
    a few cloves
    a few peppercorns
    1 bay leaf

Stick the cloves into the onion. Add onion, bay leaf, and peppercorns to stock, and simmer for 10 mins. Strain, and mix with soya milk. Melt margarine in saucepan, and mix in the flour. Cook a little, but do not allow to colour. Gradually whisk in the strained liquid, stirring to avoid lumps. Bring to boil, and simmer for a few minutes. Season with salt. If not completely smooth, run through fine sieve.

Caper Sauce

Add 1–2 Tbsp drained capers to ½ pt White Sauce. Bring to boil, and serve hot.

Fennel Sauce

Mix chopped fresh fennel into White Sauce.

Mustard Sauce

Add 2 tsp mixed English mustard and 1 tsp vinegar to ¼ pt White Sauce.

Onion Sauce

Thinly slice 3–4 oz onion. Sauté in a little margarine until transparent. Add to ½ pt White Sauce.

Parsley Sauce

Run some cold water through chopped parsley to avoid colouring the sauce and add to White Sauce.

Brown Sauce (Sauce Espagnole)   *Makes 1 pt*

  1 pt brown stock
  2 oz flour
  2 oz margarine
  1 carrot
  1 onion
  1 Tbsp tomato purée
  1 bay leaf

Fry the flour in the margarine until it is nut brown, but do not burn. Add roughly chopped onion and carrot. Gradually add the stock (hot, but not boiling), stirring out lumps. Add tomato purée, and bay leaf. Simmer for 15 mins. Strain, and use as required. (The vegetables may be used in soup or stew.)

This sauce can be kept in a refrigerator for 3–4 days. It will also keep in a deep-freeze for several weeks.

Barbecue Sauce   *Makes ½ pt*

  1 cup Sauce Espagnole
  1 onion
  1 oz margarine
  ¼ tsp cayenne pepper
  1 Tbsp crushed pineapple
  3–4 pickled gherkins
  2 tomatoes (fresh or tinned)
  1 Tbsp lemon juice

Chop the onion, gherkins, and the tomatoes. Sweat the onion in the margarine until transparent. Add all other ingredients. Bring to boil, and simmer for 3—4 minutes.

Chasseur Sauce   *Makes ½ pt*

> 1 cup Sauce Espagnole
> 1 small onion, chopped
> 1 oz sliced mushrooms
> 1 oz margarine
> 1 large tomato
> 2 tsp lemon juice
> salt, freshly ground black pepper

Sweat the onion and mushroom in the margarine. Peel and de-seed tomato, then rough-chop and add to onion and mushroom. Add Sauce Espagnole, bring to boil, and simmer for a few minutes. Add lemon juice. Season with salt and freshly ground black pepper.

Hollandaise Sauce   *Makes ¼ pt*

Real Hollandaise is a rich sauce of incomparable flavour, made from butter and egg yolk. Unfortunately, it must be strictly rejected in terms of this diet. The following recipe, however, is a surprisingly good substitute.

> ¼ pt soya milk
> 2 tsp cornflour
> salt, pepper
> 1½ oz margarine
> 2 tsp lemon juice

Boil milk, and thicken with the cornflour. Cool to blood heat. Warm the margarine to melting point, and beat into the thickened milk. Stir in the lemon juice. Season with salt and pepper.

Béarnaise Sauce

Add finely-chopped shallot, tarragon, and parsley to Hollandaise Sauce.

Apple Sauce

Peel and core some tart apples. Cut into small pieces and cook to a pulp in barely enough water to cover. Sweeten to taste with a little sugar. If too thick, balance liquid with a little water. If the apples have not been tart enough, sharpen flavour with lemon juice. If peeling and coring have been done thoroughly, there should be no need to sieve.

Bread Sauce   *Makes ½ pt*

> ½ pt soya milk
> ½ cup fresh breadcrumbs
> 1 bay leaf
> 1 small onion
> 3–4 cloves
> salt, pepper

Stick the cloves into the onion, and add to the soya milk along with the bay leaf. Bring to the boil, and simmer for 4–5 min. Add the bread crumbs, and keep hot for 20 min at the side of the stove or in a double boiler. Remove onion and bay leaf. Season with salt and pepper.

Tomato Sauce   *Makes ¾ pt*

> 1 large tin tomatoes
> 1 Tbsp tomato purée
> 1 large onion
> 1 Tbsp lemon juice
> 2 Tbsp oil
> 2 cloves garlic
> 1 tsp oregano
> salt, pepper

Chop the onion. Crush the garlic with salt. Sauté onion, garlic, and oregano in oil. Add the tomatoes and the tomato purée. Simmer until tomatoes are pulped. Pass through a sieve, or blend in a liquidiser. Balance liquid with water, or white wine. Add lemon juice. Season with salt and pepper.

Velouté

Makes ½ pt

> ½ pt chicken *or* fish stock
> 1 oz flour
> 1½ oz margarine
> salt, pepper

Melt the margarine. Stir in the flour. Add the stock (hot, but not boiling) gradually, stirring out lumps. Simmer for a few minutes to cook the flour. Season. Strain, if necessary.

"Butter" Sauce

Makes ¾ pt

Butter is one ingredient we must not use. Use of the name here is simply a convenience.

> 3 oz margarine
> 1 oz flour
> salt, pepper
> ½ pt boiling water
> 2 tsp lemon juice

Melt 1 oz margarine. Mix in the flour. Add the water gradually, stirring out the lumps. Bring to simmering point. Remove from heat. Allow to cool slightly. Add the lemon juice, and beat in the other 2 oz margarine, a small piece at a time. Keep warm, but do not boil.

Black Butter

Makes 4 oz

> 2–3 oz margarine
> 1 Tbsp vinegar *or* lemon juice

Heat the margarine in a small pan, until it starts to brown. Immediately add the vinegar or lemon juice. Take care with this operation, as the margarine is liable to "spark" when the vinegar is added.

Savoury "Butters"

The wide range of savoury butters has all but disappeared from the modern kitchen, but two remain popular. We prepare these as follows, using margarine in place of the traditional butter.

Anchovy Butter

Simply cream anchovy paste into soft margarine. The amount is not critical. Be guided by taste. Anchovy paste is very salty.

Anchovy paste used to be prepared by pounding tinned anchovies in a mortar, but tubes of anchovy paste are readily available in any food market.

Maître d'Hôtel or Parsley Butter

> juice of ½ lemon
> 4 oz margarine
> ½ cupful washed parsley
> salt

Cream the lemon juice into the margarine. Mix in the washed, chopped parsley, with a little salt. Be sure to drain the chopped parsley well, by wrapping in a cloth and squeezing as dry as possible.

If using to serve with fish "Colbert", use firm margarine. Roll to a cylinder shape in greaseproof paper, and chill to harden. It can then be sliced to represent Colbert's gold pieces (see Sole Colbert p. 72).

Mayonnaises

Soya Mayonnaise

Real mayonnaise is forbidden in this diet. It is a mixture of oil and vinegar, or lemon juice, emulsified with egg yolk. The emulsifying agent in the egg yolk is lecithin. Lecithin is also present to some degree in soya flour, which we can therefore use to replace the forbidden yolk of egg – as in the following recipe.

> 1 rounded Tbsp soya flour
> 2 Tbsp boiling water
> 4 Tbsp olive oil *or*
>   soya *or* sunflower
> 1 tsp mixed English mustard
> ½ Tbsp lemon juice *or* vinegar
> salt
> finely ground white pepper

Mix soya flour, salt, pepper, and mustard, with the boiling water. Beat in 1 Tbsp of the oil. Mix in the vinegar (or lemon juice). Beat in the remaining oil, in a thin trickle, but never pouring faster than this, otherwise the sauce may separate. Check seasoning. If a thinner sauce is required, add 1 tsp vinegar, or water.

This sauce improves by being kept overnight, and will "stand" without curdling for up to about a week. Store in a covered jar, but *not* in the fridge.

Aioli

Add 2 cloves of garlic crushed with salt to the Soya Mayonnaise.

Curried Mayonnaise

Add ½ tsp curry powder to Soya Mayonnaise. Allow to stand for 1 hour or so, in order to let flavour blend through the sauce.

Tartare, or Rémoulade Sauce

It is curious how this sauce has changed its name. Originally, Rémoulade and Tartare were two separate sauces. Rémoulade was prepared from a regular mayonnaise base, using raw egg yolk, and with the addition of capers, gherkins, and herbs. Tartare was a mayonnaise-type sauce prepared from hard-boiled yolks of egg, with the addition of chopped chives. By the 1960s, only the most up-market cookery writers were recognising the difference, and even one of these stated categorically that tartare sauce was just

Rémoulade with the addition of the chopped chives. Today, restaurants everywhere offer on their menus "Tartare Sauce", and actually serve Rémoulade. Some sauce manufacturers alter the spelling and call their product "Tartar". So do great cookery traditions gradually become eroded.

> **Soya Mayonnaise**
> capers
> gherkins
> parsley
> tarragon
> chives

Chop capers, gherkins, parsley, tarragon and chives fairly finely and mix into the mayonnaise. The quantities are not critical. A drop of anchovy essence may also be added.

An excellent Tartare Sauce can be made by using salad cream prepared with non-dairy cream (see below) in place of mayonnaise.

Salad Dressings

Non-Dairy-Fat Salad Cream

There is now a non-dairy-fat "cream" on the market. I have used it cautiously as a base for a salad cream, in small quantities, without any apparent ill-effects.

One such cream is marketed under the trade name "EQUAL" by Brooke Bond Oxo. I understand there are others.

> 2 Tbsp cream
> 2 tsp lemon juice
> 1 Tbsp water
> salt, pepper

Mix all the ingredients together. The water is necessary, because without it the cream will set like cottage cheese almost immediately.

Avocado Salad Dressing

> pulp of 1 avocado
> salt, pepper
> 1 Tbsp lemon juice *or* vinegar

Using a liquidiser, blend all the ingredients together.

Banana Salad Dressing

Follow instructions as above, substituting a banana for the avocado.

Silken Tofu

> 1 pkt tofu
> 2 Tbsp lemon juice
> salt, pepper to taste
> 2–3 Tbsp olive oil, *or* soya *or* sunflower oil

Using a liquidiser, blend the ingredients together. This makes a useful coating "mayonnaise".

Vinaigrette

> 4 Tbsp vegetable oil, pref. olive oil
> ½ tsp salt
> 1 Tbsp lemon juice *or* vinegar
> ¼ tsp pepper

Blend all ingredients together.

Sweet Sauces

Custard Sauce (with custard powder)

Proceed according to directions on packet using soya milk in place of the usual dairy milk. Note, however, that soya milk is liable to curdle, so do not try to keep the sauce hot, but serve immediately.

Sweet White Sauce

Proceed as for Custard Sauce, but thicken with cornflour.

Almond Sauce

Add a few drops of almond essence to Sweet White Sauce – but with care. Almond essence is fierce stuff!

Rum Sauce

Follow the recipe for Sweet White Sauce, but replace some of the liquid with rum: About 1 Tbsp to a ½ pt. Rum essence is *not* recommended.

Jam Sauce

Melt jam down with half its weight in water, and thicken with cornflour. Sieve if necessary.

Apricot Sauce (1)

Prepare with apricot jam, as for Jam Sauce, but thicken with custard powder.

Apricot Sauce (2)

A much superior sauce is made by liquidising tinned apricots in their own syrup and a little water, and thickening with cornflour. Stewed, dried apricots can also be used in the same way.

Lemon Sauce

Add juice and zest of 1 lemon to ½ pt boiling water. Thicken with custard powder. Sweeten to taste, and sieve.

Decorating Cream

Makes approx. ½ pt

> 2 oz icing sugar
> 2 oz margarine
> ⅓ pt cold custard *or* cornflour sauce

(Cornflour sauce can be prepared with ⅓ pt soya milk and 1 bare Tbsp cornflour.)

Beat the sugar and margarine until light and fluffy. Gradually beat in the custard or cornflour sauce (1 tsp at a time) until the mixture is of whipped cream consistency.

Quantities cannot be exact because some margarines will hold more than others.

Starters

Of the four finest starters in the world three are eminently suitable for the arthritis diet. The four are: Russian Caviare, Smoked Scotch Salmon, Native English Oysters and Pâté de Foie Gras from Strasbourg. The rich fattiness of Foie Gras rules it out absolutely for the arthritic. The other three are perfect for the diet and can be safely ordered anywhere as they are served simply with a slice of lemon and brown bread. Very expensive, but a splendid treat for a night out.

Avocado with Shrimps

Halve the avocados and remove stones. Mix shrimps with Soya Mayonnaise (p. 35) and heap on to the avocados.

Avocado with Banana

Scoop flesh from avocados, and roughly mash with a fork. Mix with an equal quantity of sliced banana and 1 tsp of Vinaigrette dressing (p. 38) per portion. Heap mixture into avocado skins. Dress with alternate slices of banana and tomato stood on edge, the tomato slices halved to match the size of the banana slices.

Avocado with Crab

Halve the avocados and remove stones. Heap with flaked white crab meat mixed with Soya Mayonnaise (p. 35). Sprinkle with paprika.

Avocado with Anchovy

Mash the avocado flesh with the anchovy oil from the tin and a little lemon juice. Pile back into skin and crisscross with anchovies thinly sliced lengthwise. Sprinkle lightly with Cayenne pepper.

Anchovy Canapés

Dress the anchovy fillets on toast in a crisscross pattern. Fill the
spaces with sliced olives, or with a star of Anchovy Butter (p. 35).
Brush the fillets with oil. Cut dressed toast slices into fingers. If the
canapés have to lie for any length of time, brush the fillets with
aspic jelly, but this adds a lot of work.

Cauliflower with Mayonnaise

Boil cauliflower florets in salted water until cooked, but still firm.
Drain, and cool.

Dress on lettuce with Soya Mayonnaise (p. 35), or with Banana
Salad Dressing (p. 38).

Cauliflower à la Grecque   *Serves 6–8 with salad*

    1 medium cauliflower (approx. 1 lb)
    juice 1 lemon *or* 1 Tbsp vinegar
    salt, pepper
    1 pt water
    8 oz tin tomatoes
    2 Tbsp olive oil

Boil all the ingredients except the oil gently, until the florets are
tender. This will take longer than usual, since the lemon juice or
vinegar hardens the cauliflower. Add oil. Reduce liquor until the
juices and oil blend. Season with salt and pepper. Cool and serve
on lettuce leaves.

Fish Pastes

Prepare from smoked mackerel, or tinned tuna, tinned salmon, or
tinned kippers. All are simply made by combining equal quantities
of fish and margarine. Drain the tinned fish free of all brine or oil,
and reduce to a paste either in a mortar or in an electric blender.

Mix thoroughly with margarine, fill into small bowls, and chill. Soft polyunsaturated margarines will not firm very well, but this will not affect the eating quality of the paste. Block margarines would firm the pastes, but being saturated fat they should be avoided.

Grilled Grapefruit

Halve the grapefruit. Sprinkle with soft brown sugar mixed with cinnamon. Grill until sugar caramelises.

Kipper

Raw

Thinly slice the kipper fillets, slanting through the flesh lengthwise. Arrange on dish, and strew with finely-sliced onion. Dress with Vinaigrette (p. 38). Serve with sliced tomato.

Tinned

Serve kipper fillets straight from the tin in own oil with a lettuce and tomato salad. Tinned kipper has an excellent flavour.

Melon Boats

Cut melon into wedges, and remove seeds. Cut the flesh into inch cubes, leaving these *in situ* on the slice. Sprinkle with chopped preserved ginger, or serve with ginger sugar (1 Tbsp caster sugar mixed with ½ tsp ground ginger).

Melon with Parma ham

The superb way to serve melon is with Parma ham, but, initially in this diet, ham is not allowed. It may be cautiously tried once complete mobility and absence of pain have been achieved.

Mushrooms à la Grecque   *Serves 4–6 with salad*

½ lb mushrooms
1 onion
2 Tbsp olive oil
¼ pt water
juice 1 lemon
8 oz tin tomatoes
salt, pepper

Slice the onion and sweat with the mushrooms in the oil. Add water, lemon juice, and tomatoes. Season with salt and pepper. Simmer, and reduce liquor until the juices blend with the oil. Cool.

Serve on lettuce with sliced tomato.

Shrimp Cocktail

Mix shrimps with Soya Mayonnaise (p. 35), or with avocado flesh blended in a liquidiser with a little lemon juice.

Dress on shredded lettuce in a melba dish, or in a goblet.

For Shrimps Marie Rose, add 1 tsp of tomato purée or ketchup.

Smoked Mackerel

Smoked mackerel has established itself, in recent years, as a firm favourite. It is hot-smoked, so needs no further cooking. Slice or flake it.

Serve it simply with a slice of lemon and brown bread.

It can also be sprinkled with onion, and Vinaigrette dressing (p. 38), and served as a salad with lettuce and tomato.

Smoked Salmon

An aristocrat of starters, smoked salmon should be served simply with a wedge of lemon and thinly sliced brown bread.

Tuna

Tinned in Brine

Drain, and slice or flake on to lettuce. Dress with Vinaigrette (p. 38) and sliced tomato.

Tinned in oil

Treat as above; or flake and treat as for Shrimp Cocktail (p. 44).

Crudités and Savoury Dips

Crudités

> raw carrot
> turnip
> celery
> cucumber
> fennel
> peppers
> large white radish

Cut into sticks about 3 inches long and ¼-inch across.

Also, for dipping: Anchovy Straws, Melba Toast, and Potato Matchsticks (see below).

Anchovy Straws

Mix anchovy paste with a sprinkling of Cayenne pepper into a short pastry mix. Pin out to ¼-inch thickness, and cut into straws about 3 inches long. Tray up, and cook in a moderate oven. Be careful not to burn.

Melba Toast

Make slices of toast, then split them. Cut into fingers, and toast the soft underside. Alternatively, brown triangles of very thinly cut bread on a wire in moderate oven.

Potato Matchsticks

Cut raw potato into large matchsticks. Wash, drain, and dry in a towel. Deep-fry in vegetable oil till crisp. Do not add salt until matchsticks are cold.

Avocado Dip

Blend the avocado flesh with lemon juice and a little salt and pepper. Pile back into the half shells of avocado, or into goblets, and chill. Should be prepared as near to serving time as possible, to avoid discoloration.

Banana Dip

Mash bananas, and mix with Soya Mayonnaise (p. 35).

Curried Mayonnaise Dip (See p. 36)

Lentil, or Chick Pea Paste

Blend a piece of fresh ginger root in a liquidiser with a little of the cooking liquor of lentils or chick peas. Add the cooked lentils or chick peas, and blend to a paste, adding cooking liquor as necessary. May also be prepared with Soy sauce or Worcestershire sauce in place of the ginger.

Peanut Butter

Blend peanut butter with a little Soya Mayonnaise (p. 35) and Cayenne pepper to taste.

Tahini

Similar to peanut butter, but made from sesame seed, this is available from health food shops. Mix the tahini paste with an equal amount of water, a squeeze of lemon juice, and a little vegetable oil – preferably olive oil. Some brisk mixing will be necessary to start with. Alternatively, just mix with water, and then blend in some Soya Mayonnaise (p. 35).

Tomato Dip

Drain all liquid from a tin of tomatoes, and blend the tomatoes in a liquidiser with a little lemon juice and Worcestershire sauce. Season lightly with salt, and mix in (without blending) a little chopped oregano, or tarragon.

Serve chilled.

Soups

Bean Soup

    4 oz butter beans
    1 large onion
    1½ oz margarine
    2 pt any stock
    salt, pepper

Soak the beans overnight. Roughly chop the onion, and sweat in
the margarine. Add the beans and the stock, and cook until the
beans break down. This will take at least 2 hrs. Blend in a
liquidiser, or pass through a sieve. Season with salt and pepper,
only when process is complete, because salt hardens the beans,
and they then take longer to cook.

A pressure-cooker will reduce the overall time to about 15
mins; but be careful not to burn, because a pressure-cooker
evaporates water at a frightening rate. Balance liquid with boiling
stock or water to desired consistency.

Flageolet beans will give a soup of a delicate green colour, and
will take less time to cook.

Cauliflower soup

    1 small cooked cauliflower
    1 large onion
    2 oz margarine
    1½ oz flour
    1½ pt chicken stock
    ½ pt soya milk
    parsley

Chop the onion finely, and sweat in the margarine. Mix in the
flour, and gradually stir in the hot, but not boiling, stock. Be
careful to stir out lumps. Blend the cauliflower with the soya milk,
in a liquidiser; or press through a sieve. Add to soup. Simmer for 5
mins.

Sprinkle in a little parsley before serving.

Celery Soup

Proceed as for Cauliflower Soup, using the leaves and trimmings
of a head of celery. The water the celery is cooked in may be used
as stock. The chopped green of celery leaf may be used to replace
parsley.

Chicken Broth with Rice   *Serves 4*

> 2–4 oz cooked chicken, free of fat and diced
> 2 pt chicken stock
> 1 large carrot
> 1 large onion
> 1 oz margarine
> 4 oz rice
> ½ Tbsp chopped parsley
> Salt, pepper

Finely chop the carrot and onion and sweat them in the margarine. Add the rice, and stir over a low heat until the margarine is
absorbed. Add the stock. Season, and boil until rice is soft. Add
the diced chicken, and simmer for a few minutes to thoroughly
heat the chicken. Stir in chopped parsley immediately before
serving.

Cream of Chicken Soup   *Serves 4*

> 4 oz cooked chicken
> 1½ pt chicken stock
> 1 finely chopped large onion
> 2 oz margarine
> 2 oz flour
> ½ pt soya milk
> ½ Tbsp washed chopped parsley
> salt, pepper

Sweat the onion in the margarine until transparent. Mix in the
flour, and cook a little, but do not brown. Add the stock (hot, but
not boiling) gradually, while stirring to avoid lumps. Bring to boil,
and simmer for 10 mins. Shred the chicken, and add to the soup
with the soya milk. Season. Simmer for 2–3 mins.

Note: With white soups or stews, chopped parsley should be well washed under running water; otherwise, it will colour the dish.

Cock-a-Leekie

This was a favourite soup in old Edinburgh. The old recipes suggest that it was more of a leek and chicken stew, than a soup. Controversy raged about whether or not it should be served with prunes. It was originally prepared by boiling an old fowl with large pieces of leeks; but, as we must remove all fat, we have to adapt.

Prepare as for Cream of Chicken soup, but use 4 good-sized leeks in place of the onion. Remove the tops of the leeks and discard, leaving about half the green. Split the leeks lengthwise, and wash thoroughly. Chop the leeks into 1-inch lengths. The soup will have to be simmered for a longer period, in order to cook the leeks. If you wish to add prunes, Edinburgh fashion, soak them well until they are plumped. Cook in the soup with the leeks.

Serve two or three prunes per plate.

Chicken and Sweetcorn Soup

Proceed as for Cream of Chicken soup, but blend ½ of 8 oz can of sweetcorn with the soya milk, and add to the soup.

Stir in the other ½ of the can of sweetcorn, unbroken, with the diced chicken. Simmer for 5 mins, to heat through.

Lentil Soup   *Serves 4*

    4 oz lentils
    1 large onion
    1 large carrot
    1 oz margarine
    2 pt any stock
    1 bay leaf
    salt, pepper

Roughly chop the onion and carrot, and sweat in the margarine. Add the lentils, and stir over the heat for a minute or so until the margarine is absorbed. Add stock and bay leaf. Cook for about 1 hr until lentils have completely broken down. As with beans, salt lengthens the cooking time, and so season after the lentils are cooked. Remove bay leaf. Pass through a sieve, or electric blender. Serve with "sippets" (¼-inch cubes of bread browned in hot oil, and drained on kitchen paper).

A pressure-cooker reduces the time required for the whole process to about 10 mins, but beware of burning.

Minestrone   *Serves 6*

    4 oz dried haricot beans
    2 pt any stock
    1 large onion
    1 carrot
    1 small turnip
    2 sticks celery
    1 oz cabbage
    ½ lb fresh tomatoes (or small tin)
    2 oz peas frozen or fresh
    2 oz macaroni or spaghetti
    2 cloves garlic
    ½ tsp oregano
    ½ Tbsp chopped parsley
    salt, pepper

Soak the haricot beans overnight. Drain and wash. Add to stock and simmer for 2 hrs. Chop the vegetables fairly finely, and sweat in the margarine. Add to stock and beans. Add peas, and roughly-chopped tomatoes. Cook till vegetables are tender. Add macaroni, oregano, and crushed garlic. Cook for further ¼ hr. Season with salt and pepper. Add a little water if necessary, but soup should be almost thick enough to stand a spoon in.

Stir in chopped parsley just before you serve.

Mulligatawny

Method 1   *Serves 4*

>   1 large onion
>   1 cooking apple
>   2 oz margarine
>   ½ Tbsp curry powder
>   1½ oz flour
>   2 pt any stock
>   1 oz long grain rice
>   1 Tbsp desiccated coconut
>   2 cloves garlic
>   juice ½ lemon
>   salt

Finely chop the onion and cooking apple, and sweat in the margarine with the curry powder. (Be careful not to burn.) Mix in the flour. Add the stock gradually, stirring out lumps. Bring to boil. Add the rice and coconut. Cook till rice is tender. Crush the garlic with salt, and add to the soup with the lemon juice. Season with salt.

More curry powder may be added if you like it hot.

Method 2   *Serves 4*

This makes a superior and fresher-tasting soup.

>   1 large onion
>   1 cooking apple
>   2 pt any stock
>   2 oz margarine
>   ½ inch fresh root ginger
>   2 cloves garlic
>   1½ oz flour
>   1 tsp ground cumin
>   ½ tsp ground coriander
>   ½ tsp ground turmeric
>   ¼ tsp cayenne pepper
>   ¼ tsp freshly ground black pepper
>   1 oz long grain rice
>   ½ Tbsp lemon juice
>   salt

Finely chop the onion and cooking apple. Liquidise the root ginger with about a cup of the stock. Fry the spices and finely-chopped garlic in the margarine for 1 min. Add the onion and apple, and sweat till transparent. Add the flour, then stir in the stock and the blended ginger. Bring to the boil. Add the rice, and simmer till the rice is tender. Add the lemon juice, and season with salt.

Mushroom Soup   *Serves 4*

>   1 medium onion
>   2 oz margarine
>   2 oz flour
>   1½ pt stock
>   4 oz white button mushrooms
>   ½ pt soya milk

Finely chop the onion, and sweat in the margarine until transparent. Add the flour. Add the hot stock, stirring to avoid lumps. Finely slice the mushrooms and throw into the soup. Simmer for a few minutes. Add the soya milk. Boil for 1 min.

Note: With older mushrooms, parboil them first with just enough water to cover, and a squeeze of lemon. This will prevent discoloration.

White Onion Soup

Proceed as for Cauliflower Soup (p. 48), using ½ lb onions to 2 pt liquid. Add 1 clove of garlic crushed with salt.

Brown Onion Soup   *Serves 2–3*

>   ½ lb thinly-sliced onions
>   2 oz margarine
>   1 bay leaf
>   1 pt brown vegetable stock *or* yeast extract stock
>   1 clove garlic
>   salt, pepper

Brown the onions in the margarine, but be careful not to burn.

Add the stock and bay leaf. Crush the garlic in salt, and add to soup. Boil gently for 5 mins. Season.

Serve with croutons (toasted slices of French bread, or rolls).

Green and Yellow Split Pea Soup

Proceed as for Lentil Soup (p. 50).

Potato and Leek Soup   *Serves 4–6*

1 lb peeled potatoes
4 good-sized leeks
2 oz margarine
2 pt any stock
salt, pepper

Chop the potatoes into ½-inch dice. Wash the leeks well and cut into ½-inch pieces. Sweat the leeks in the margarine. Add the potatoes, and the stock. Bring to the boil, and simmer for about 1 hr or until the potatoes have broken down. Season with salt and pepper.

Potato and Carrot Soup   *Serves 4–6*

1 lb peeled potatoes
2 large carrots
1 large onion
2 oz margarine
2 pt any stock
salt, pepper

Cut potatoes into ½-inch dice. Grate or finely shred the carrots. Roughly chop the onion. Sweat the onion in the margarine. Add potatoes, carrots, and stock. Cook until the potatoes have broken down. Season with salt and pepper.

Scotch Broth   *Serves 4–6*

    2 oz pearl barley
    2 oz dried marrowfat peas
    2 pt stock
    1 large carrot
    equal weight of swede
    1 large onion
    2 leeks
    2 oz cabbage *or* kale
    2 oz margarine
    1 Tbsp chopped parsley
    salt, pepper

Soak pearl barley and peas overnight. Drain and wash. Add to the stock, and simmer for 1 hr. Grate or finely chop the vegetables, and add with the margarine, to the soup. Simmer for one more hour, or until the peas are tender.

Serve sprinkled with chopped parsley.

Note: Scotch Broth actually improves by being cooled and reheated the following day; but be sure to bring to the boil and simmer for at least 10 mins before serving. One thing I have seen passed off as Scotch Broth and which is emphatically not so, is consommé garnished with lumps of vegetables. As with Minestrone, this soup should be almost thick enough to allow a spoon to stand upright in it. With a hunk of bread, it is a meal in itself.

Tomato Soup   *Serves 4*

Method 1

    1 lb ripe fresh tomatoes *or* 1 large tin tomatoes
    1 large onion
    1 Tbsp vegetable oil
    1 pt any stock
    1 tsp oregano *or* thyme
    1 bay leaf
    ½ Tbsp sago
    salt, pepper
    1 tsp sugar (optional)

Rough chop the onion, and fry in the oil until transparent. Add the tomatoes, and cook till pulped. Add the herbs and stock, and simmer for 10 mins. Pass through a sieve to remove tomato skins and seeds. Return to pan, and bring to boil. Sprinkle in the sago, stirring to avoid lumps. Cook until sago is transparent. Season with salt and pepper. Sweeten, if liked, with sugar.

Method 2   *Serves 4*

> 1 lb ripe fresh tomatoes *or* 1 large tin tomatoes
> 1 onion
> 1 carrot
> 2 oz margarine
> 1½ oz flour
> 1 pt any stock
> 1 bay leaf
> ½ tsp dried oregano
> salt, pepper

Chop the onion and carrot, and fry in margarine until the onion is transparent. Add the flour. Add the hot (but not boiling) stock, stirring to avoid lumps. Add tomatoes and herbs. Bring to boil, and cook until the carrot is soft and the tomatoes completely broken down. Pass through a fine sieve, or blend in the liquidiser. Return to pan, and simmer for 5 mins. Season with salt and pepper.

Cold Soups

Gazpacho   *Serves 3–4*

> ½ pt tomato juice
> 1 clove garlic
> ½ cucumber
> 1 onion
> 1 green pepper
> 4 Tbsp olive oil
> 2 Tbsp lemon juice
> 3–4 tomatoes
> salt
> freshly ground black pepper

Blend in a liquidiser the tomato juice, the garlic, ¼ the cucumber, ½ the onion, and ½ the green pepper. Chill in refrigerator. Chop into small dice the remaining ¼ cucumber, ½ onion, green pepper and the tomatoes.

Mix into the chilled soup, together with the olive oil and the lemon juice. Season, and serve.

Vichyssoise   *Serves 4*

> ½ lb potato
> 2 large leeks
> green tops from 2 sticks of celery
> 2 oz margarine
> 1½ pt white stock
> ½ pt soya milk
> 1 doz chopped olives
> salt, pepper

Chop the potato, leeks, and celery fairly finely. Cook with margarine in the stock until just tender. Blend in liquidiser. Stir in soya milk. Garnish with chopped olives. Cool, and chill in refrigerator.

Fish

This is the perfect source of protein for our diet. Today, the fishmonger offers us a wider variety of fish than ever before. Modern transport gets fish to the fishmonger's slab in any part of the country, in good condition. Modern fishing techniques enable us to buy, in any supermarket, fish that has been frozen marble-hard within minutes of leaving the water. Our ever-increasing preference for holidays abroad introduces us to fish, and fish dishes, that few would have even looked at otherwise.

Even so, fried haddock and chips is still the best-selling dish in any cafeteria; and provided that it is fried in vegetable oil, this means that there will always be a dish suitable for our diet available in almost every catering establishment. It will not be perfect. The cooking oil will be mostly a blend of vegetable oils such as rape seed, and coconut, neither of which is as high in polyunsaturates as we would like. The breadcrumbs used for dressing the fish will contain "permitted colouring" and "permitted preservatives", neither of which is desirable.

We can be pretty certain, however, that the fish will not be egg-washed. Only the most up-market establishments use egg-wash nowadays, and they are the kind of place where you can explain your requirements, and have them satisfied in every detail. In such establishments, they are more likely to be offering grilled Dover sole and salmon, rather than haddock and chips; but even so, such dishes as Whole Sole "Colbert" are egg-washed, bread-crumbed, deep-fried, and served with Maître d'Hôtel butter. One must still be careful!

Fresh-water fish such as carp, perch, and pike, are rarely available through the fishmonger; but angling is by far the most popular participation sport in this country, and a lot of "coarse" fish goes to waste. If there is no angler in the family, there is almost certainly one living in your vicinity. Gifts of game fish such as salmon and trout may be too much to expect, but a surprising number of anglers just do not bother to bring home coarse fish, simply because they do not know anyone who eats them.

Cooking Methods

Grilling

The simplest method of cooking fish, and also the one which brings out its finest flavour. The difficulty most people experience with grilling is in attempting to turn the fish on a wire grill, or even in the grill pan. The problem is easily overcome. Use a thick-based frying pan, or skillet. Heat the pan with a thin covering of oil or margarine. Place the fish in the pan and cook over heat for a minute or two. Put the pan under the grill and brown the fish. It will then be cooked – and without any intermediate handling.

Charcoal Grilling/Barbecue

For this purpose, a special double wire is available and may be obtained in any good hardware store. Charcoal grilling is considered by many to be the supreme method of cooking fish. The fish is simply floured, brushed with oil, seasoned with sea salt, placed between the double wires, and grilled on both sides until the flesh comes away easily from the bone. Large fish should be deeply slashed several times on each side to facilitate the cooking process. Enthusiasts throw a handful of aromatic herbs on to the charcoal halfway through the cooking process, to give an exotic flavour to the fish. (Charcoal is not hot enough until it begins to show white ash.)

Boiling

This word, for me, conjures up pictures of great fish-kettles steaming in Victorian kitchens for poorhouse dinners. I wonder how many generations of school children have shared my consequent aversion to boiled fish, and have had to be re-educated? I prefer the expression "poached". See under "Poaching".

Baking – Method 1

Oven temperatures and cooking times depend on the size and shape of the fish. Thin flat fish will cook faster than thick round fish. As a general guide allow 10–15 minutes for each pound and cook light thin fish at 425°F and heavier fish at 400°F (see oven chart on p. 159).

Baking – Method 2

Large fillets, or whole fish, are wrapped in foil and baked in the oven. An older, more rustic version of this method, is to wrap whole fish, such as trout, gutted and seasoned with salt, in a sheet of newspaper. Wet the newspaper, and cook the parcel in the oven until the paper is dry. The fish will then be cooked. The skin will stick to the paper and will be removed when the fish is unwrapped. This is a method also employed by the gypsy, and by the hill fisherman. They use a thicker wrapping of newspaper than for an oven, and cook the parcel in the embers of an open fire.

Deep Frying

Suitable for thin fillets or small whole fish. Fish is normally egg-washed and bread-crumbed, but as egg-wash is made from whole egg, we cannot use it for this diet. Either use egg white only, or batter made from flour and water to coat the fish before crumbing. White of egg, however, is somewhat expensive to use because twice as many eggs are required; and, as the yolk cannot be used, it will be wasted.

Batter for coating is simply made with plain flour and water mixed to the consistency of single cream. Shop-bought "fish dressing" contains several additives, and is better avoided.

Fresh bread produces a crumb which is too large, does not stick well to the batter, and absorbs too much cooking oil. Crumbs should be made from dry, stale bread, finely ground. A liquidiser will produce breadcrumbs in seconds, but in its absence, a fine crumb can be produced by pounding very dry bread with a rolling-pin.

Dust the fillets in seasoned flour. Lightly coat with egg-white or flour and water batter. Pass through breadcrumbs. Shake off surplus crumbs and fry in deep oil at a temperature not less than 375°F (190°C). When the fish float, they are cooked.

The other deep-frying method is to fry in batter, "à la chip shop", or "à l'Orley". The fish-shop batter is made simply with plain flour and water mixed to the consistency of double cream. The Orley batter is a little more complicated, and is prepared as follows.

Orley batter

To coat 4 large or 8 small fillets

4 oz plain flour
½ Tbsp oil
1 egg white
¼ pt water

Mix flour, water and oil to a smooth batter. Beat the white of egg stiffly and fold gently into the batter.

Fish fried in batter, especially using Orley batter, must be served immediately as it goes quickly soggy.

Shallow-Frying

Breadcrumbed fish can be fried in this way, but it is not recommended. The fish is very easily burned, and it usually absorbs too much fat, as the uppermost side is always at a lower than optimum frying temperature.

Meunière Style. Dip the fish in seasoned flour and fry in polyunsaturated margarine, or in oil. When frying in margarine, the margarine must be heated to the point where all the watery content has evaporated; but beyond this point, the margarine burns very easily, and so care must be taken.

Poaching

This should be done with just enough liquid barely to cover the fish. If the fish is lost in pints of water, it will be tasteless.

Smear a dish with margarine. Lay on the fish, and just cover with water. Cover with greaseproof paper. The steam thus contained will ensure that any exposed part of the fish is completely cooked.

If additional liquid is required for making sauce, use a fish stock prepared from fish bones.

Bass

Sea bass is a handsome fish with an elegant shape and shining silver scales. The firm white flesh, also, has an excellent flavour; but unfortunately this fish is all too seldom seen on the fish-monger's slab. Its average weight is 2–2½ lb, which makes it a suitable size for baking (p. 59). Alternatively, before baking, stuff with some chopped onions and herbs.

Barbecue grilling

Bass is an ideal fish for charcoal grilling on a barbecue (p. 59). Make several deep slashes across both sides of the fish. Sprinkle with salt, and brush with oil. Do not have grill too close to the coals, otherwise the outer skin may be badly burned before the fish is cooked. Extra flavour may be added by throwing some rosemary or fennel on to the grill a minute or so before the fish is completely cooked.

Bream

Fresh-water bream

Treat as carp (p. 63).

Salt-water bream

The fillets on the fishmonger's slab may be bream but are more likely to be the Norwegian red fish, Berghylt, which is oilier and firmer than cod but of a good flavour. Cook as for cod (p. 63). It should be cheaper than cod, and I prefer it.

Brill

Brill closely resembles turbot (p. 74) and should be poached or baked in the same way. It is however smaller than turbot, more delicate and fragile, and should be poached or baked whole. If you do not possess a special fish kettle, use a large frying-pan or roasting tray for poaching.

Carp

Large carp should be baked (p. 59). Allow 15 min per 1 lb. Small carp may be filleted and fried Meunière style (p. 61).

Carp are farmed in ponds in Germany as trout are in the U.K. There they fry them in deep fat in a crisp batter, chip shop style (p. 60), which I have found to be delicious. They are then served with salad, dressed German-style, which is much sharper than French dressing or Vinaigrette because of the much higher vinegar content. This balances beautifully the rich oiliness of the fish.

Cod

Poached with Parsley Sauce

Take individual-sized cod fillets or steaks cut in 4–5 oz pieces and place in a margarined skillet or ovenware dish just large enough to hold the fish in a single layer. Season with salt, and add enough water barely to cover the fish. Cover with oiled greaseproof paper. Bring gently to the boil, and simmer until fish is opaque – about 6–7 mins. Alternatively, once fish has been brought to simmering point, place in a hot oven for 10–12 mins.

Make a Velouté (p. 34) with the liquid strained from the fish and a little soya milk.

Add 1 dstsp washed, chopped parsley. Dish the fish, and dress with the sauce.

Grilled Cod Steaks

See Grilling (p. 59).

Baked Cod Steaks

Dip the steaks into seasoned flour. Brown quickly on both sides. Place on foil. Sprinkle with chopped basil, chopped parsley, and a squeeze of lemon juice. Envelope the foil, and bake in moderately hot oven for 20 mins.

Cod Steaks Baked Portuguese Style

As above, but add some finely-sliced onion and de-seeded, chopped tomato.

Salt Cod

Although salt cod has been very widely used throughout history, today it has almost disappeared from the fishmonger's slab and is very much a minority taste.

Soak the fish overnight, wash off, then poach in fresh water for 10–15 mins. Drain, and discard water.

Proceed as for fresh cod (see above). One method popular in Italy is to bake in an ovenware dish with chopped onion, chopped tomato, parsley, and basil, with 2–3 Tbsp of water or white wine. Surround with sliced, parboiled potatoes, cover, and bake for about 30 mins in a moderately hot oven.

Coley

Also known as saithe, pollock, or coalfish, it is similar in flavour to haddock, or whiting, and is cheaper than either. The snag is that there is a black marbling running through the flesh, and this lends it an unattractive appearance when poached. But deep-fried in batter or breadcrumbs and served with a slice of lemon or with Rémoulade Sauce (p. 36), it is every bit as good as whiting or haddock. Coley is also excellent for fishcakes.

Conger Eel

The tough flesh of this fish makes it unsuitable for the usual grilling, frying, or poaching processes, but it is eminently suitable for Fish Stews (p. 80), and dishes such as Paella (p. 111).

Dabs/Flounders

Grill, poach, or fry, as for sole (p. 72) or plaice (p. 70). Dabs and flounders are the poor relations of the flat fish family, but discriminating people recognise that, when these fish are absolutely fresh, they are at least the equal of their more expensive cousins.

Eels

Eels are excellent for the diet; but people tend either to love eels or hate them. If you love them, buy them jellied or smoked from your fishmonger. See also recipe for Matelote (p. 83).

Grayling

Bake, fry, or grill, as trout (p. 74).

Haddock

Whole haddock, with its characteristic mark of "St Peter's thumb-print", is very easily distinguished from the otherwise similar whiting and codling. Filleted, however, it is difficult indeed to distinguish from the other two. You will have to depend on your fishmonger for this – although it doesn't matter all that much, as the eating quality is very similar. The best method of cooking is to fry it either in breadcrumbs or in batter. Serve with either lemon or Rémoulade Sauce (p. 36).

Finnan (Findon) Haddock

This is whole haddock split and smoked on the bone. It gets its name from the village of Findon in the north-east of Scotland, where the process was invented. The very expensive smoked salmon always excepted, it is undoubtedly the finest of the smoked fish range. Poach it in a little soya milk with a nut of margarine. Serve it in the milk, with bread or plain boiled potatoes.

Smoked Fillet of Haddock

The process of smoking is different from that used for Finnan Haddock, and some of the flavour of the fish is thereby lost. Cook as Finnan Haddock.

The use of artificial dyes in the smoked fish industry has heretofore been common practice, but smoked fish free of dye is now gradually becoming available. It is worth building up public demand by asking for this.

Hake

Hake may be treated as cod (p. 63). Although not so commonly available as it once was, it is a firm-fleshed fish that responds well to baking, or grilling, and should be bought whenever the opportunity arises.

Halibut

Cookery writers love to refer to halibut as "the Queen of fish" – salmon being the "King". It is undoubtedly the finest fish caught in our northern seas, and is priced accordingly. Large halibut is best cut into steaks and grilled, or baked. If it is small enough, it may be baked whole, as brill (p. 62), or small turbot (p. 74); but these smaller "chicken" halibut just don't have much flavour. Small "chicken" halibut are better filleted and fried Meunière style (p. 61).

Halibut steaks also poach well, and may be served with any sauce recommended for fillet sole (p. 72).

Herring

Over-fishing a few years ago almost completely deprived our tables of these fine fish; but strict control of catches has fortunately made them available again. They are probably still the cheapest protein flesh one can buy, and one of the best in food value.

Fried

Boned, split herrings may be simply seasoned, dipped in flour, and fried; but I think that the Scottish method of frying them in oatmeal is infinitely preferable. Sprinkle the boned herring with salt, and coat with fine oatmeal (coarse oatmeal falls off, and that which stays on absorbs too much cooking fat). Cook quickly in hot vegetable oil in a frying-pan. Coolish oil will penetrate both the oatmeal and the fish.

Very small herrings may be left whole and cooked in this way.

Grilled

Use whole, gutted fish. With a sharp knife, make three shallow slashes across the back to facilitate cooking. Dust with seasoned flour. Brush with oil. Grill on both sides for about 5 mins. Serve with Mustard Sauce (p. 31).

Soused Herring   *Serves 4*

> 4 large or 8 small herrings
> a few peppercorns
> 1 bay leaf
> 1 medium onion
> equal quantities of water and vinegar to cover
> ½ tsp salt

Remove heads and tails from gutted herrings. Pack them tightly in an ovenware dish. Sprinkle with a few peppercorns, 1 bay leaf and some thinly-sliced onions. In a separate pan, boil equal amounts of vinegar and water in quantity sufficient to cover the fish. Season the water/vinegar with salt, and pour over the fish. Cover with foil and bake in a moderate oven for about 20 mins. Cool in the cooking liquid. Serve cold with a salad.

Boned, split herrings can also be cooked in this manner. Roll them from the head end down. Again, so that they retain their shape, pack tightly in an ovenware dish.

Kippers

These are smoked, split herrings. Unfortunately, as with Smoked Haddock, they are usually artificially dyed; but again, it is possible to obtain the undyed variety, and it is worth asking for it. The dyed kipper is easily recognisable by its dark copper-brown colour, in contrast to the undyed kipper which has a golden-brown appearance.

The most popular method of cooking kippers is to grill them – but do not put them on a wire. Lay them in the grill pan with a knob of margarine and 1 Tbsp of water. They need only be cooked on one side. Frying is not advised, mostly because the taste of kipper stays with the pan.

The kipper smell can also permeate the house – although it is possible to use various stratagems to reduce the possibility of this happening. One such is to put the kippers head down into a tall jug, and to fill the jug with boiling water. Leave for 5 mins, drain and serve. The flavour of kipper is strong enough to ensure that this will still make a palatable dish.

Ling

The flesh of ling is similar to that of cod, although somewhat coarser. The flavour is much the same. Large quantities of ling are caught but not much reaches the fishmonger's slab. Presumably it goes into processing for fish fingers, or is exported. Its elongated, almost eel-like shape, gives it one advantage over cod. It cuts into even-sized steaks for the greater part of its length. The steaks are best baked, and served with a Velouté Sauce (p. 34). Flour and season the steaks, and place them in a margarined baking dish. Dab them with margarine, and pour 2 Tbsp water round them – not over them. Bake in a hot oven. Remove the steaks, and deglaze the tin with a little water. Use the essence thus obtained, cohered with a roux (p. 27), for the Velouté.

Mackerel

Mackerel is a fish which has gained enormously in popularity in recent years. Not so long ago, our fishermen caught them mainly for export. Little boys, catching them by the dozen with a large hook with a feather attached, couldn't give them away for cat's food. But times have changed. We now know what our fellow Europeans have always known – that the rich, oily flesh of the mackerel is wonderful food. It is also perfect for an arthritis diet.

Grilled Mackerel

Mackerel may be grilled either whole or filleted.

To grill whole, make three deep slashes across the back. Flour and season. Brush with oil. Grill for 6–7 mins each side, dependent on size.

Filleted mackerel should be grilled for about 5 mins. Serve as herring, with a Mustard Sauce (p. 31). Parsley Sauce (p. 31), Fennel Sauce (p. 30), or Maître d'Hôtel "butter" (p. 35) are also recommended.

Gooseberry Sauce is an old-time favourite for serving with grilled mackerel. The sharpness of green gooseberries offsets the rich oiliness of the mackerel. Some recipes suggest making a purée of the gooseberries, sweetened with sugar, as served with goose or pork. More interesting, perhaps, is to use gooseberries in a Velouté, as grapes are used in Sole Véronique (p. 73). Halve some hard green gooseberries and parboil until just tender. Drain, and fold into a Fish Velouté (p. 34), taking care to avoid breaking the gooseberries.

Soused Mackerel

Prepare as for Soused Herring (p. 67), but allow 30 mins' cooking time.

Smoked Mackerel

Unlike kippers and smoked haddock, smoked mackerel is prepared by a hot process, so that the flesh comes to us cooked. It is simply sliced or broken, and served with a salad – usually as a starter.

Baked Mackerel with Tomato

Pack in ovenware dish as for sousing. Sprinkle with thinly-sliced onion and sliced tomato. Add 1 bay leaf, and just cover with tomato juice. Dot with margarine. Season with salt. Cover with foil and bake in a moderate oven.

Monkfish

The monkfish is actually the "angler" fish, the greater part of which consists of head and mouth. Only the tail is used and it makes excellent eating, either in Fish Stews (p. 80) or served as "scampi". At one time, fishermen threw the whole fish away, simply because nobody wanted it, but then commercial cooks discovered that it made very good "scampi"; and so long as this knowledge was kept within the trade, monkfish tail remained very cheap. A few years ago, however, a TV personality let the general public in on this secret, and within weeks, the price of monkfish tail had trebled. Nevertheless, it is still cheaper than prawns, which is what true scampi are.

"Scampi"

Cut monkfish fillets into thin strips about 2 ins long. Dust these with seasoned flour, and fry in deep fat. Serve with a wedge of lemon, or Rémoulade Sauce (p. 36). The scampi can be "bulked up" by coating before frying, either in batter (p. 61), or batter and breadcrumbs.

Pilchards

These once-plentiful fish have all but disappeared from the fishmonger's slab, but are still fished for in Cornwall and the south-west.

About the size of the Portuguese and Mediterranean sardine, they are every bit as delicious. Make sure that they are perfectly fresh. Grill them simply with a sprinkling of sea salt. The flesh is oily enough to make brushing with oil unnecessary.

Plaice

Small whole plaice are best grilled.

Fillet plaice is usually fried in breadcrumbs, and served with lemon, or with Tartare Sauce (p. 36).

Fillets of plaice may also be used in any of the recipes for Poached Sole (p. 72), but plaice flesh is fragile, and so handle carefully.

Large plaice may be baked, as turbot (p. 74) or brill (p. 62); but the flesh is so fragile that transferring the fish from baking dish to serving dish can be tricky. An oven-to-table type of dish may be the answer.

Salmon

Salmon is expensive, but still cheaper than fillet steak, and there is almost no waste. Salmon is so good in itself that it needs no *cordon bleu* recipe. Simply grill or poach the steaks. Serve grilled steaks with a piece of lemon, or Maître d'Hôtel "butter" (p. 35).

Whole salmon, or larger pieces to serve cold, should be poached in a "Court Bouillon" (p. 28). Boil the carrot, onion, bay leaf and peppercorns for 5–10 mins in a quantity sufficient to cover the salmon amply. Add the vinegar and salt. Add the salmon and bring slowly back to simmering point.

Allow to simmer for only 3–4 mins. Withdraw pan from heat, and leave the fish to cool in the liquid overnight. The flesh will pick readily away from the bones, and the skin will be easily removed.

Slice cold salmon in head to tail direction, with a sharp knife. It is very difficult to cut across the grain, and any attempt to do so will probably end up with broken fish. Serve with Soya Mayonnaise (p. 35) or Silken Tofu (p. 38).

Pickings from cooked bones and head of salmon make excellent fish cakes.

Skate

Poached

Just cover skate wings with salted water. Add 1 Tbsp vinegar. Bring to boil, and simmer until the bone separates readily from the flesh – about 20 mins. Serve with Caper Sauce (p. 30) or Black Butter (p. 34).

Fried

Skate should be boiled before frying, and therefore the process is a bit tedious. Fried skate is popular, however, with some people. Cook the skate wings in salted water, but *not* until the flesh starts to fall away from the bone. About 15 mins should be enough. Drain thoroughly on a cloth. Sprinkle with flour, and shallow-fry, or dip in batter and deep-fry. Serve with lemon, or Tartare Sauce (p. 36).

Sole

Some cookery books give over 400 different recipes for sole, but mostly these recipes refer to sauces and garnishes to serve with the four basic methods: grilling, frying, poaching, and baking.

The dark skin of sole is always removed before cooking. Many people consider it criminal to serve a Dover sole other than whole, and grilled for preference. The less favoured lemon and megrim soles are treated and served as Dover sole.

Grilled

See grilling (p. 59). Serve simply with a wedge of lemon.

Fried

Lemon and megrim sole fillets are often fried in breadcrumbs or in batter in the same way as fillet plaice (p. 60). For cooking in batter, use the Orley style batter (p. 61), and serve with Tomato Sauce (p. 33).

Fried goujons

Cut the sole fillets into little-finger-sized pieces. Batter and breadcrumb, and fry in deep oil. Serve piled in a heap with a piece of lemon, or Rémoulade Sauce (p. 36).

Colbert

This is the best-known version of frying whole in breadcrumbs. Colbert was a Treasurer of France, and the idea is to represent a purse full of gold coins. Run a knife down the spine, on the skin side, and roll the flesh back to the edges of the fish, but do not detach. Break the backbone at both ends and in the middle, to make its removal easier when cooked.

Coat with batter (p. 60) or egg white and breadcrumbs. Fry to a golden brown in hot deep fat, remembering to keep the rolled flesh held back. Remove the backbone, and serve with a few slices of Maître d'Hôtel "butter" (p. 35) placed in the cavity.

Poached

This is served classically with a fish glaze, reduced with white wine, mounted with butter, and/or Béarnaise Sauce; but for our purposes, served with a Velouté Sauce (p. 34) made with fish stock or with fish stock and white wine. Out of several hundred styles of serving, a few of the more popular are as follows.

Bonne Femme

Coat with a Fish Velouté (p. 34) mixed with finely-chopped shallots, sliced mushrooms, and chopped parsley.

Aux Crevettes

Coat with a Fish Velouté (p. 34) mixed with shrimps. Tinned or frozen shrimps are quite suitable, but wash the shrimps well before mixing into the sauce. Otherwise, with tinned shrimps, the flavour of the brine will permeate the sauce, and with frozen shrimps the taste of these might otherwise prove rather too strong for the delicate flavour of the sole.

Dugléré

Coat with a Fish Velouté (p. 34) mixed with finely-chopped shallots, skinned and de-seeded diced tomatoes, and chopped parsley.

Véronique

Coat with a Fish Velouté (p. 34) and peeled muscat grapes. There are two methods. In Method 1, the grapes are cut in half and deseeded, mixed in with the sauce, and served hot. In Method 2 the fish is coated with the Velouté, the grapes are chilled and sprinkled over the dish immediately before serving. This second method provides an interesting contrast of texture and flavour between the chilled grapes and the hot fish.

Shallow-Frying

Meunière

See under Shallow-Frying (p. 61).

Serve garnished with a few slices of lemon which have had the skin removed, and Black Butter (p. 34).

Trout

Salmon may be "the King of fish" but there are some anglers who maintain that they would not eat it in preference to a good brown trout, or a not too large fresh run sea-trout. The trout we are likely to encounter in the fishmonger's is farmed rainbow trout. These may not rival wild trout in flavour, but still make very good eating.

Trout may be grilled, or fried Meunière style (p. 61). Large trout may also be baked in foil.

Trout Amandine (with almonds)

Cook small trout whole, but fillet larger trout, and prepare as for Meunière (p. 61); but fry the almonds in margarine until the margarine is coloured, then add lemon juice. Pour over the trout.

Small Brook or "Burn" Trout

Simply dust with seasoned flour and fry quickly in shallow fat. A better method to my mind, however, is to dip them in fine oatmeal and fry Scotch style, like herrings (p. 66).

Turbot

Turbot is a very fine but somewhat expensive fish. It is one of the few white fish that are really suitable for serving cold. It should be poached as salmon (p. 71), and served with Mayonnaise (p. 35); but do not chill, because the gelatinous nature of the flesh makes it somewhat rubbery if it gets too cold.

Small turbot may be baked whole in an open dish or in foil. They may also be poached – see brill (p. 62). Large turbot are cut into steaks, and grilled or poached.

Whitebait

Wash the whitebait, and toss in a towel to remove surplus water. Place the whitebait in a plastic bag with a handful of seasoned flour, and shake until the fish are coated. Fry in deep oil until crisp. Heap them on a dish and serve with a wedge of lemon.

Devilled Whitebait

Mix dry mustard and cayenne pepper into the flour. Continue as above.

Whiting

Whole whiting is easily distinguished from haddock. It is slimmer, and does not carry the mark traditionally known as "St Peter's thumb print". When filleted and skinned, however, it is very difficult indeed to distinguish from small haddock.

Popular at one time in forms such as "curled whiting" (curled head to tail, breadcrumbed and fried in deep oil), whiting seems nowadays never to appear on restaurant menus. Nevertheless, there seems always to be a great deal of "haddock" around. One wonders! When whiting is fresh, it is quite as good as haddock, but it very quickly goes stale. Filleted, but with the skin left on, it is known to the trade as "wet cutlets", and in that form is used mostly by fish and chip shops. The fact of these having a good turnover means that they can indeed serve the fish in the required fresh condition. Their product fried in vegetable oil is enjoyed throughout the land, and is perfectly suitable for the diet. For home consumption, prepare as haddock (p. 65).

Shellfish

Crabs

Unless you are totally familiar with crabs, it is best to buy them cooked from a fishmonger. It is difficult, otherwise, to ensure freshness.

Dressed Crab

Remove the claws. Hold all the legs together, and pull off. The gills and guts will come with them. Remove the soft, yellowish-brown flesh from the shell. Set aside. Break off the shell to the dark line running round it about ½ inch from its edge. Wash the shell thoroughly, scrubbing the outside with a nailbrush until it is shining-clean.

Mix the soft flesh from the inside of the shell with breadcrumbs and a little Worcestershire sauce, and salt, and pile into the shell.

Crack the claws and legs with a blunt instrument, and extract the meat. If you can get the meat in the tips of the claws out whole, put this aside for decoration. Flake the rest of the white meat, and pile on top of the dark meat mixture.

Decorate with parsley and the claw tips, also shredded anchovy, using this last item in place of the traditional hard-boiled egg. Serve with Vinaigrette dressing (p. 38).

Cockles

These are rarely sold raw; but if you are fortunate enough to live within reach of an uncontaminated beach, cockles may be treated as oysters and eaten raw, provided they are absolutely fresh.

They are easier to open than oysters. Take two cockles, fit the hinge of one to the hinge of the other, and twist. They may also be cooked as mussels (p. 77).

Fried from raw

Remove from shell. Dry in a cloth. Fry in batter (p. 60) in deep oil. Serve with a wedge of lemon, or Rémoulade Sauce (p. 36).

Fried from cooked

Coat in batter (p. 60), and breadcrumb. Fry in deep fat. Serve with a wedge of lemon, or Rémoulade Sauce (p. 36).

Lobster

This is one for the "night out" or the expense account lunch; but do remember that most of the traditional recipes are totally unsuitable for this diet, relying heavily as they do on ingredients such as cream, and cheese. Stick to plain grilled lobster which, in any case, is one of the best ways of cooking this fish. Either that, or order cold lobster with salad.

Mussels

Moules Marinières   *Serves 2*

> 2 pt well-washed mussels
> 1 small onion
> 1 oz margarine
> ½ cup water *or* white wine
> Beurre Manié (p. 27)

Rough-chop the onion, and sweat in the margarine. Add the water/wine. Throw in the mussels. Tightly cover, and cook rapidly for 4–5 mins, or until mussels are open. Set mussels aside. Reject any which haven't opened, strain liquid to remove any sand. Thicken liquid with Beurre Manié and reheat to just below boiling.

Serve mussels in their shells in soup plates with the cooking liquor poured over them.

Oysters

Serve raw on the half-shell with lemon and thinly sliced brown bread and polyunsaturated margarine. Some establishments serve tabasco sauce or ground black pepper with the oysters but it is not recommended. Allow at least 6 oysters per person.

In the not-so-far-off days when oysters were cheap they were cooked in dozens of different ways on their own or added to all kinds of pies and puddings. Now they are much too expensive for such usage.

Fish Concoctions

Fish Pie   *Serves 4*

I do not think that fish goes well with pastry, but fish pie with pastry seems to be popular in certain areas, and very firm-fleshed fish such as conger eel and rock salmon (dog fish) which require stewing can be used to advantage in this way.

1 lb fish	water to cover
1 medium onion	salt, pepper
1 bay leaf	puff pastry (p. 148)

Stew the fish with onion and bay leaf. Make a Velouté Sauce (p. 34) with the stock, and fold in the roughly-broken fish. Season to taste. Turn into a pie dish and allow to cool. Cover with puff pastry made with vegetable fat and cook in a hot oven until the pastry is ready – about 20 mins.

An easier and more popular method is to cover with mashed potato, shepherd's pie style. Brush the top with melted margarine, and brown in a hot oven. The shepherd's pie style, to my mind, produces a much happier marriage of flavours.

Fish Cakes   *Serves 2*

These can be made from almost any kind of fish, including tinned salmon, and tinned tuna, also smoked fish such as smoked haddock and cod. I personally prefer the stronger flavour of the smoked fish.

½ lb cooked fish
½ lb boiled potato
1 oz margarine
salt, pepper
Batter
4 oz flour
¼ pt water

Mash the potatoes with the margarine; and mix thoroughly with the cooked fish, salt and pepper. Shape the mixture into 4 cakes, and cool thoroughly. Dust the cakes with flour. Coat with batter and breadcrumbs. Fry in hot oil until brown.

If using tinned fish, make sure it is thoroughly drained before mixing with the potatoes.

Salt cod makes a flavoursome fish cake, but takes more trouble to prepare. Soak the salt cod overnight in water, and rinse thoroughly in fresh water, before boiling. Salt cod will take much longer to cook than fresh fish. Allow about 15 mins. Mix as above, but do not add further salt to the mixture.

Kedgeree   *Serves 4*

(Quantities are variable but the following is a guide)

> 6 oz long grain rice
> 8 oz flaked cooked fish
> 1–2 oz margarine
> salt, pepper

Boil the rice in salted water until just tender. Do not overcook.
Drain, and mix in the margarine. Fold in the fish, and season.

This is a very simple dish, which is prepared in the time taken to
cook the rice – around 10–15 mins. Both rice and fish can be
cooked previously, and then re-heated, but the extra trouble of
re-heating and the little time saved scarcely make the exercise
worth while.

I prefer the flavour of smoked fish, such as haddock or cod, and
tinned salmon or tuna also make a flavoursome kedgeree.

Fish Savoury   *Serves 2*

This can be prepared with smoked haddock, kippers, or tinned
tuna.

> 4 oz smoked haddock *or* other fish
> 1 oz margarine
> 1 oz flour
> ¼ pt soya milk
> ¼ pt water
> 1 tsp chopped parsley
> cayenne pepper

Poach haddock or kipper in a mixture of water and soya milk.
Remove skin. In the case of tinned tuna, drain off oil or brine, and
bring to boil in the milk and water mixture. Make a roux (p. 27)
with the margarine and the flour. Add the cooking liquid from the
fish, stirring out lumps. Simmer for 2–3 mins. Break, but do not
mash, the fish and fold into the sauce. Add parsley. The mixture
should not require seasoning with salt.

Serve piled on toast. Sprinkle with Cayenne pepper.

Tuna Fish Pie
Serves 2

> 1 × 7 oz tin tuna
> 1 large onion
> 1 oz margarine
> 1 small tin chopped tomatoes
> freshly ground pepper
> salt
> 1 lb (approx.) mashed potatoes

Slice the onion and sweat in ½ the margarine and the oil drained from the tuna fish. Add the tomatoes. Flake the fish, and fold into the onions and tomatoes. Add pepper. Check salt. Cover with mashed potatoes. Smear with melted margarine. (Spread with a hot knife.) Heat through and brown in a hot oven (15–20 mins).

Fish Stews

Bouillabaisse
Serves 4 generously

There is a mystique about Bouillabaisse that the French have been careful to cultivate and that has elevated it from its humble origins to haute cuisine and a very high price on the menu! It is no more haute cuisine, in fact, than steak and kidney pudding or Irish stew. It was originally a poor man's dish, made by Mediterranean fishermen from any part of their catch that would not sell in the market. All French recipes call for *rascasse*, and that is the one fish we cannot get here. The other fish, however, are all obtainable in this country, although varieties like John Dory and Conger Eel are not always easy to find. The selection of fish used varies with the hundreds of different recipes, but the following list includes most of them.

haddock	conger eel
sea bream	John Dory (the French St Pierre)
lobster	gurnard
prawns	eel
crab	whiting
bass	mullet

The one ingredient that all consider to be essential is saffron. It would be fair to say, in fact, that without saffron the dish would not be Bouillabaisse, but it would still be a delicious fish stew – and saffron is very expensive. You will require per person, ½–¾ lb fish on the bone. If you get your fishmonger to trim off head, tail, and fins, be sure to take these with you to use for the stock.

> 3 lb mixed fish on the bone (traditionally John Dory,
>   gurnard and conger eel, but any combination from
>   the above list)
> 3 onions
> 2 Tbsp oil (pref. olive)
> 2 cloves garlic
> 3 peeled and deseeded tomatoes
> 1 glass white wine (optional)
> pinch dried saffron
> sprig of parsley
> 1 bay leaf
> sprig of thyme
> salt

Make a fish stock with the fish heads and trimmings, and the herbs. Chop the onion, crush the garlic with salt, and sweat in the oil. Add the chopped tomatoes. Cut the fish into 3-inch lengths, and lay on top of the onions and tomatoes. Add the saffron, and wine. Add enough strained fish stock to just cover the fish. Season with salt. Bring to the boil, and simmer for 15 mins. Check seasoning. Serve with slices of toasted French bread.

In the Eastern Mediterranean they boil potatoes and carrots in the fish stock, and these are served whole with the fish. Other recipes suggest that potatoes cut in ½-inch-thick slices should be cooked with the fish. Either method makes the Bouillabaisse a single-dish meal.

Chowder

Chowder is arguably more a soup than a stew, but under whatever classification, it is still a substantial dish. Any New Englander will tell you that an essential ingredient of Clam Chowder is salt pork – but don't believe this. We can prepare an excellent chowder without it. We can prepare an excellent chowder, in fact, without clams!

Smoked Haddock Chowder   *Serves 4–6*

    1 lb smoked haddock fillet
    1 lb peeled potatoes
    1 large onion
    2 oz margarine
    1 Tbsp flour
    ½ cup soya milk
    1 Tbsp chopped parsley
    cream crackers
    salt

Cover the haddock with water, and cook. (This will take only a
few minutes.) Cut potatoes and onions into ½-inch dice, and
sweat in the margarine. Stir in the flour. Add the liquid that the
haddock was cooked in, and just enough further water to cover
the potatoes. Cook until the potatoes are tender. Break the
haddock into bite-sized pieces, and mix into the soup. Whiten
with a little soya milk, but do not boil further. Season, and
sprinkle with parsley.

   Serve with broken crackers.

Mussel Chowder   *Serves 4–6*

    1 qt mussels thoroughly washed and scrubbed
    ½ pt water
    ½ pt white wine
    1 lb peeled potatoes
    1 large onion
    2 oz margarine
    1 Tbsp flour
    ½ cup soya milk
    1 cup chopped parsley
    salt
    cream crackers

Bring to the boil water or ¼ pt water and ¼ pt white wine. Throw
in the mussels. Cover tightly with a lid and boil fiercely for about 5
mins. The mussels should then be cooked, but check that they are
all open. If any fail to open, remove and throw away. Remove the
mussels from their shells, and strain the cooking liquor.

   Note: It is advisable to strain the liquor through a cloth, since
there may be some grains of sand coming out of the mussels.
Proceed as for Smoked Haddock Chowder (see above).

Clam Chowder

Where fresh clams are available, proceed as for Mussel Chowder (see above). Fresh cockles and scallops can also be prepared in the same way, but the scallops will require to be cut into pieces. Tinned clams are a very good substitute for the fresh variety. Tinned clam juice also enhances the flavour of any of the chowders.

Matelote   Serves 4–6

Matelote is the fresh-water fish equivalent of Bouillabaisse. It is prepared from a mixture of any fresh-water fish, especially carp, pike, and eel, or any single one of these. Purists would certainly not agree, but firm-fleshed salt-water fish like conger eel or monkfish also make a fine Matelote.

> 2 lb fish
> 1 large onion
> 2–3 shallots
> 2–3 cloves garlic
> 3 Tbsp margarine
> 2 Tbsp oil
> 2 Tbsp brandy (optional)
> ½ bottle red wine
> water as required
> 1 Tbsp flour
> 2 oz button mushrooms
> chopped parsley
> croutons

Cut the fish into bite-sized pieces and chop the onion and shallots. Crush the garlic. Sauté fish, onion, shallots and garlic in the oil and 1 Tbsp margarine. When the fish pieces start to brown, flame them in the brandy (if used). Add the wine, and enough water to cover. Season, and cook gently till the fish is tender. Sauté the mushrooms in the remaining 2 Tbsp margarine. Stir in the flour, and cook for a few minutes without allowing to colour. Mix in the liquid from the fish, stirring out lumps. Balance liquid with stock, or water, to make a slightly-thickened sauce. Stir in the lemon juice and the fish pieces. Sprinkle with parsley.

Serve very hot, with fried croutons.

Poultry

After fish, poultry is going to be our most useful flesh. Frozen supermarket poultry should be avoided if possible, because in the freezing process sodium polyphosphate is added to help the meat absorb water. This alone is undesirable, but also our food should be as free as possible from added chemicals. A frozen product free of sodium polyphosphate is now appearing on the market, and is very clearly labelled. It is a little more expensive than the water-added variety – but still cannot be more extravagant than water sold at the price of poultry meat!

Frozen chicken is especially unsuitable for sauté chicken dishes for example, because bacteria can lurk in unthawed parts, and the short cooking process involved may not be enough to sterilise.

Only young, fresh birds should be used. Boiling fowls carry too much fat. And as the skin of poultry is heavily impregnated with fat, it should always be discarded by anyone on our diet. Sometimes, as in the case of roast chicken, it may simply be removed from the cooked flesh; but in other dishes, you must remove the skin before cooking, so that the fat will not permeate the whole dish.

Chicken

Boiled Chicken

Serves 4–6

> 1 × 3 lb chicken
> 1 onion
> 1 stick of celery *or* green from 1 head
> 1 small carrot
> 1 bay leaf
> salt, pepper

Remove any layer of fat from just inside the bird. Cover the chicken and other ingredients with water. Season and cook till tender (about 1 hr). Lift from the stock, remove skin, and skim stock completely free of fat.

Use for dishes such as fricassée, risotto, à la King, etc. If not for immediate use, leave the skin on to prevent the flesh drying out.

The best way to remove fat from stock is to allow the stock to cool completely, then simply lift off the solidified fat.

Note: "Boiling Fowl" is not as good as chicken for boiled chicken dishes. It is initially cheaper per pound to buy, and the flavour is stronger; but the carcase contains a large amount of fat, and the proportion of bone is higher, so that the cost of cooked edible flesh per pound is considerably greater than that of chicken. The very much longer cooking time required, also, means an increase in fuel costs; added to all of which, the flesh becomes very dry.

Chicken Burgers

Serves 2–3

8 oz raw chicken
4 oz breadcrumbs
1 onion
1 Tbsp oil
1 tsp mixed herbs
1 egg white
salt, pepper

Mince the chicken. Chop the onion finely. Mix herbs and seasoning through the breadcrumbs. Mix in the oil. Add chicken, onion and egg white, and combine thoroughly. Divide into 4 or 6. Shape into burgers. Pass through breadcrumbs. Fry in shallow oil.

Serve with Chasseur Sauce (p. 32).

Chicken Casserole

Serves 4

Any part of the chicken can be used for this dish, but I think that chicken thighs are the most suitable.

8 chicken thighs
1 Tbsp oil
1 Tbsp margarine
1 large onion

1 carrot
1 Tbsp flour
12 oz tin tomatoes
1 tsp oregano
1 clove garlic
1 glass red wine (optional)
salt, pepper

Skin the chicken thighs, and dust with flour. Brown the thighs in the oil and margarine, in a heavy-based casserole. Remove, and set aside. Chop the onion, carrot, and garlic, and fry till they start to colour. Stir in the 1 Tbsp flour. Add the tinned tomatoes and oregano. Return the chicken pieces to the casserole, and add sufficient water to just cover the chicken. If preferred, some of the water may be replaced by red wine. Bring to the boil, cover, and simmer for 40–45 mins till tender.

This is an ideal dish for slow cooking in the oven, or in a slow cooker.

Chicken Cutlets   *Serves 2*

½ lb left-over chicken
1 oz margarine
½ oz (1 Tbsp) flour
¼ pt chicken stock
1 shallot *or* small onion
salt, pepper
batter (p. 60)
breadcrumbs
oil for frying

Chop the chicken fairly finely. Chop the onion very finely. Sweat onion in the margarine. Mix in the flour. Add chicken stock. Stir out lumps. Bring to boil and cook for 2–3 mins. Mix in the chicken and seasoning, and boil for another minute or so to heat the chicken thoroughly – but be careful not to burn. Turn mixture out on to a tray and allow to cool. When quite firm, shape into cutlets. Coat with batter and breadcrumbs, and fry in deep oil.

Serve with Tomato Sauce (p. 33).

Curried Chicken

Serves 4

Method 1

>8 chicken thighs
>2 oz margarine
>1 onion
>1 tart apple
>1 Tbsp flour
>2 tsp curry powder
>½ pt any stock
>½ Tbsp desiccated coconut
>½ Tbsp chutney
>1 Tbsp lemon juice
>salt

Flour the chicken joints and brown in the margarine. Remove, and set aside. Chop the onion and apple, and sweat in the margarine. Stir in flour and curry powder. Cook for a few minutes. Add the stock, and stir free of lumps. Add all other ingredients. Add salt to taste, and simmer until chicken is tender.

Serve on boiled rice.

Note: cooked chicken can be used for this dish.

Method 2

Serves 4

This will produce a superior curry which is much nearer in flavour to real Indian curry.

>8 chicken thighs *or* equivalent
>2 oz margarine
>½ tsp turmeric
>½ tsp coriander
>½ tsp cumin
>½ tsp chilli powder
>1 tsp poppy seed
>2 chopped medium onions
>4 chopped tomatoes
>1 crushed clove garlic
>1 inch fresh ginger root
>soya milk as required
>salt
>2 Tbsp water to blend ginger

Brown the chicken joints in the margarine. Remove, and set aside.
Fry the spices in the margarine for ½ min. Add the onions, and
sweat until transparent. Add tomatoes, and the liquidised ginger.
Add chicken joints. Moisten further as necessary with soya milk,
or a little water. Season with salt. Simmer till tender.

Serve on boiled rice.

Fried Chicken

Fried in batter

> *Batter*
> approx 4 oz plain flour
> approx ¼ pt water

Skin the chicken joints and dip in seasoned flour to help the batter
to stick. For the batter, mix flour and water to the consistency of
double cream. Dip chicken in the batter, and coat evenly. Drop
into deep oil. Fry till brown and crisp. Serve with Barbecue Sauce
(p. 31), or Tomato Sauce (p. 33).

Fried Chicken Maryland   *Serves 4*

> 4 boneless chicken breasts (supremes)
> 2 Tbsp margarine
> 2 Tbsp oil
> 2–3 oz breadcrumbs
> salt, pepper, flour
> batter coating (see above)
> 2 bananas
> 1 sm. tin sweetcorn

Dust the chicken with seasoned flour. Coat thinly with flour and
water batter, or with white of egg. Pass through breadcrumbs.
Shallow-fry in a mixture of margarine and vegetable oil.

Serve with fried banana, sliced horizontally, and with *sweetcorn patties* which are made as follows. Mix a little flour
into tinned creamed sweetcorn to make a batter of dropping
consistency. Season with salt. Fry.

Chicken Fricassée
Serves 4

12–16 oz cooked chicken
¾ pt chicken Velouté (p. 34)

Mix bite-sized pieces of boiled chicken with a Velouté made with the chicken stock. If preferred, some of the chicken stock may be replaced with soya milk. Heat thoroughly, but if soya milk is used, do not boil.

Chicken à la King

Prepare as for Fricassée. Serve on plain boiled rice, or on risotto rice. Garnish with strips of blanched and skinned red peppers. Using tinned peppers (pimento) saves a lot of effort.

Chicken and Mushroom Pie
Serves 4

8 chicken thighs
1 onion
½ bay leaf
4 oz button mushrooms
2 oz margarine
flour to thicken
salt, pepper
puff pastry (p. 148)

Skin the chicken pieces, chop these in half, and place in a pan with just enough water to cover. Add the bay leaf and the rough-chopped onion. Season, and simmer till the chicken is tender (approx. 30 mins). In a separate pan, sweat the mushrooms in the margarine, and mix in the flour. Stir in ½ pt of the stock from the chicken, to make a Velouté (p. 34). Add the cooked thighs and simmer for 2–3 mins. Turn into a pie-dish, and allow to cool.

When quite cold, cover with puff pastry (p. 148) and allow to rest for 15 mins. Brush the pastry with white of egg or soya milk. Mark a pattern of diamonds on the pastry with a sharp knive, but do not cut through. Cook in a moderate oven until pastry has risen and is nicely browned – approx. 20–25 mins. Note: The pastry must rest before being placed in the oven, or it will shrink. Shrinking will also take place if the pastry is used to cover hot food.

Rappie Pie

Serves 6, or 4 gluttons

Here is a curious recipe from Nova Scotia. The word "Rappie", I believe, is a child's version of "rapture". The original ingredients include bacon and butter, but we can prepare the dish without these.

> 1 × 3 lb chicken
> 2 large onions
> 1 bay leaf
> 3 lb potatoes
> 2 oz margarine

Boil the chicken with the onions and bay leaf in enough water to cover for about 1 hr, till tender. Season with salt and pepper. When cooked, separate the meat from the bones, and keep hot. Grate the potatoes. Place in a cloth bag and squeeze out every drop of water into a receptacle. Measure this water and mix an equal amount of boiling broth from the chicken into the grated potatoes. Do this into a pan large enough to allow for vigorous stirring. The broth should be added slowly, stirring the while to avoid lumps. Keep over the heat, and continue stirring like mad until the potatoes take on a jelly-like appearance. Put half the potatoes in the bottom of a well-margarined pie-dish. Cut into pieces the chicken and onion drained from the broth, and spread over the potato. Top with the rest of the potato mixture. Dab with margarine, and cook in a hot oven for 1½–2 hrs until a brown crust has formed.

Serve with Apple Sauce (p. 33).

Risotto

Serves 4

> 12 oz cooked chicken
> 1 onion
> 2 oz margarine
> 1 large cup long grain rice
> 3 cups stock
> ¼ red pepper
> ¼ green pepper
> 1½ oz green peas

Chop the onion and sweat in the margarine until transparent. Add the rice, and stir until the grains are well coated. Add the stock, and simmer. After 10 mins, add the chopped peppers, with the peas, and the chicken cut into small pieces. Continue simmering until all the stock has been absorbed.

Alternatively, the chicken pieces can be mixed with Velouté (p. 34) and served over the rice.

Roast Chicken

Roast the chicken, using vegetable oil for basting. Allow 20 mins per lb for small birds. Set oven at 400°F, reduce after 5 mins to 375° (see Oven Chart on p. 159); Allow 15 mins per lb for birds 6 lb or over. Start at 400°F, reduce temperature to 350°F. If the bird is browning too rapidly, reduce heat and cover with foil. When cooked, remove skin, and serve with clear gravy made from the roasting-tray essences which have been skimmed of all fat. Do not stuff the bird because, even if stuffing is prepared with margarine or vegetable oil instead of suet, chicken fat from the skin will penetrate the stuffing.

Parsley and thyme, or chestnut, or any other stuffing prepared with margarine, can be cooked separately, either baked or steamed in foil.

Stuffing for Roast Chicken   *For 1 average chicken*

> 1 oz margarine
> 2 oz breadcrumbs
> 1 finely chopped small onion
> ½ Tbsp self-raising flour
> ½ tsp chopped thyme
> 1 tsp chopped parsley
> 1 egg white
> water
> salt, pepper

Melt the margarine, and mix well into the dry ingredients. Add the white of egg and just enough water to make into a not-too-firm paste. Roll in a sheet of well-margarined grease-proof paper, and bake beside the chicken. Alternatively, the stuffing can be steamed in a pudding basin.

The stuffing can be varied by adding almonds, chopped cooked apricots, apple, chestnuts, hazel-nuts, or any other such ingredient.

Sauté Chicken

With Almonds   *Serves 4*

> 8 chicken thighs *or* 4 breasts, skinned and boned
> flour to coat
> 1 onion
> 1 Tbsp sliced almonds
> ½ Tbsp flour
> 1 cup tomato juice
> 1 glass white wine *or* water
> salt, pepper

Flour the portions (chop breasts in two) and fry in the oil until golden brown. Remove, and set aside. Sweat the onion and almonds in the pan. Mix in the flour. Add the tomato juice and wine (or water), stirring till smooth. Season, and simmer. Add the chicken. Continue simmering gently for 20 mins, or till tender, depending on size of chicken portions.

With Apricots   *Serves 4*

Use the same ingredients as for Sauté Chicken with Almonds, substituting 1 small tin apricots for the almonds. Proceed as for above, omitting the almonds and holding back the addition of the apricots until the chicken is cooked. Cut the apricots in half, and add to the dish, simmering just long enough to heat through.

This recipe also works especially well with turkey breasts.

Chicken Bonne Femme   *Serves 4*

> 8 chicken thighs *or* 4 breasts skinned and boned
> flour to coat
> 4 oz spring onions *or* 1 rough chopped onion
> 4 oz potato cut in ½-inch dice
> 1 Tbsp oil
> ½ Tbsp flour

2 oz button mushrooms
½ pt chicken stock
salt, pepper

Flour the chicken and brown in the oil. Remove and set aside. Sweat onions, potatoes, and mushrooms, in the oil. Mix in ½ Tbsp flour. Moisten with chicken stock. Season to taste. Add chicken portions. Simmer gently for a further 20 mins or until tender.

Chicken Chasseur

Serves 4

8 chicken thighs *or* 4 breasts
flour to coat + ½ Tbsp flour
½ Tbsp oil
1 large chopped onion
2 oz sliced mushrooms
1 small tin tomatoes, chopped
1 cup chicken stock, lemon juice

Skin the chicken, flour, and brown in the oil. Remove and set aside. Add the ½ Tbsp flour to the oil, and cook to a nut brown. Do not allow to burn. Add the onions and mushrooms, and stir in the chopped tomatoes. Stir in the chicken stock, and the lemon juice. Season. Simmer for a few minutes. Add chicken, and simmer for a further 20 mins or until tender. Serve sprinkled with chopped parsley.

Stoved Chicken

Serves 4 generously

4 chicken legs
2 lb potatoes
1 lb carrots
½ lb onion
4 cooking apples
2 oz margarine
salt, pepper
1 cup stock *or* water

The amount of vegetables indicated could accommodate 2 more legs and so could easily stretch to 6 smaller portions.

This is a very old dish and originally was cooked over an open fire. Stoved means stewed and it can be cooked in a thick based pan or casserole either on top of the stove or in the oven.

Skin the chicken legs and remove any fat. Joint them. Slice the potatoes ½ in thick. Cut the carrots, onions, and cooking apples into somewhat finer slices and keep separate. Fry the chicken legs in the margarine for a few minutes, then remove from casserole. Place the ingredients in separate layers in the casserole, sprinkling each layer with salt and pepper, and finish with a layer of potatoes. Add a cup of stock, or water. Bring to simmer, cover tightly, and cook very slowly for 1½ hours. Shake occasionally to prevent sticking.

Chicken Liver

Chicken livers will probably be tolerated by anyone following this diet, but should only be tried cautiously at first.

Be sure in every case that the gall bladders have been completely removed from the liver. Any trace of gall will make the livers taste horribly bitter and they will be almost inedible.

Devilled Chicken Liver   *Serves 2*

> ½ lb chicken liver
> 1 oz margarine
> Worcestershire sauce
> cayenne pepper
> made mustard
> 1 cup Brown Sauce (p. 31)
> salt
> chopped parsley

Cut each liver in two, and sauté in a little margarine until just cooked. Prepare a Devilled Sauce by adding Worcestershire sauce, Cayenne pepper, and made mustard to Brown Sauce. Bring sauce to boil, add livers, and simmer for 1–2 mins. Add seasonings to taste in the quantities you can tolerate.

Serve on a bed of plain boiled long-grain rice. Sprinkle with parsley.

Chicken Liver Pâté

½ lb chicken livers
1 small onion
1 clove garlic
3 oz margarine
½ tsp mixed herbs
salt, pepper

Chop the onion, and sweat with the chicken livers and garlic in 1 oz of the margarine. Do not allow the liver to brown, or it will form a crust which will give a gritty texture to the pâté. When the livers are cooked, add the herbs and seasoning. Mix to a smooth paste in a liquidiser or food processor. Allow to cool. When quite cold (but not chilled) mix in the remaining margarine until it is completely integrated with the paste. Pack into small pots. Make airtight with a little melted margarine poured on top of each. Chill in the refrigerator. Do not freeze. Freezing and defrosting again produce a gritty texture in the pâté. The pâté can be kept in a fridge for up to a week.

Note: Use fresh herbs for preference as dried herbs often contain undesirable bits of stalk.

Chicken Liver Risotto   *Serves 2–3*

½ lb chicken livers
2 oz margarine
1 chopped onion
1 clove chopped garlic
1 cup long grain rice
2 cups any stock
salt
pepper

Cut the livers into four, and fry in the margarine until pink inside. Remove and set aside. Sweat the onion and garlic in the margarine remaining in the pan. Add the rice, and stir to coat the grains with margarine. Add stock and seasoning, and simmer until the liquid is absorbed and the rice is tender.

Fold the liver into the rice. If well-cooked liver is preferred, return the liver to the pan with the stock, and simmer with the rice; but this does make the texture of the liver dry and grainy.

Chicken Liver Vol-au-Vents

Vol-au-Vents cases

Prepare with puff pastry recipe (p. 148). Roll pastry out to about ⅜-inch thickness. Rest for 20 mins. Cut out 3-inch rounds. With smaller cutter cut out an inner round but only go about half-way through the pastry. Rest for 20 mins. Brush with white of egg. Cook in a hot oven for 15–20 mins. Before cooling, run knife round inner ring. Remove inner round and use to cap the Vol-au-vent when filled. Scoop out soft inside of the vol-au-vent and discard.

Vol-au-Vents filling   *Fills 2 × 3-inch cases or 4 small bouchets*

> ½ lb chicken livers
> ¼ lb mushrooms
> 1 cup Brown Sauce (p. 31)
> 1 Tbsp margarine *or* oil
> ½ red pepper

Cut the livers and the pepper into ½-inch dice. Slice the mushrooms. Sauté the liver in a little margarine or oil. Remove and set aside. Sweat the mushrooms and pepper in the pan, and moisten with Brown Sauce. Bring to the boil. Add the liver, and simmer without boiling for 2–3 mins. Fill into vol-au-vent cases.

Duck

Farmyard duck is absolutely taboo for this diet. At least fifty per cent of the weight of such birds is fat of the kind we most want to avoid.

The fat of wild creatures, however, is different in chemical composition from that of the farmyard variety. In addition to this, very little fat is contained in their flesh, and so wild duck may be tried cautiously. But even then, make sure that the portion served is free from fat, and that every scrap of skin has been removed.

Wild duck, traditionally, is simply roasted and served with an orange salad.

Game Birds

The flesh of game birds may be cautiously tried since being creatures of the wild, they are likely to contain less fat than domestic birds.

All young birds may be simply roasted. Salt them, and keep them well basted with margarine. Cook in a hot oven. Smaller birds, such as partridge, will take about 25 mins. Grouse will take about 35 mins, and pheasant about 45 mins to 1 hr. A large cock pheasant, past its first youth, will take even longer. If it becomes apparent that the cooking process will have to be prolonged, wrap the bird(s) in foil to finish cooking. This will keep the flesh moist, and prevent burning. Older birds should be casseroled as Pigeon (see below).

The silly practice of hanging game till putrefaction has begun is no longer fashionable. Game should be hung for only a few days to allow *rigor mortis* to relax. Wild duck should be cooked as soon as possible.

Pigeon

Young birds may be roasted as game birds. Older birds are better casseroled.

Casserole Pigeon   *Serves 4*

    4 pigeons
    2 Tbsp oil
    1 carrot
    1 similar sized piece of turnip *or*/and parsnip

1 Tbsp flour
3 cups any stock
½ Tbsp tomato purée
¼ lb mushrooms (optional)
1 small tin tomatoes (optional)
salt, pepper

Dredge the pigeons with flour, and fry them in the oil until browned all over. Remove from pan, and set aside. Chop the vegetables and add them with 1 Tbsp flour to the oil. Fry till flour is light brown. Stir in the stock to make a light sauce, replacing some of the stock with red wine, if preferred. Add tomato purée. Season with salt and pepper. Return birds to pan. Cover, and simmer till birds are tender.

Mushrooms and tinned or fresh tomatoes can also be included among the vegetables if desired.

Turkey

Roast Turkey

Set oven at 425°F (see Oven Chart, p. 159). Brush turkey with oil and sprinkle with salt. Place on roasting rack in oven. After 5 mins reduce temperature setting to 350°F. Allow 15 mins per lb. Allow extra 20 mins over for small bird. Turn and baste occasionally. Don't be concerned if turning is difficult. It is desirable but not absolutely necessary. Cover bird with foil if browning too rapidly.

Fillets of Turkey Breast

These may be treated as *schnitzel* or *escalope*. Sprinkle the breasts with water, and place them between two sheets of plastic (a plastic shopping bag is ideal). Beat them out to about ¼ inch thick, then dip them in seasoned flour. Coat with white of egg or batter, and then with breadcrumbs. Shallow fry in oil.

Escalope Napolitaine

Serve with spaghetti and Tomato Sauce (p. 33).

Wiener Schnitzel

Serve with a garnish of anchovy and capers, and a quarter lemon. (The traditional recipe for this garnish includes yolk of hard-boiled egg; but this, of course, cannot be included here.)

Zigeuner Schnitzel

Serve with Chasseur Sauce (p. 32), plus shredded red and green peppers.

Turkey Breast Olives   *Serves 4*

> 4 turkey breast fillets
> Risotto filling (see below)
> 2 Tbsp oil
> 1 onion
> 1 Tbsp flour
> 1 small tin tomatoes, chopped
> ½ pt any stock
> salt, pepper

Cut turkey breast fillets in half. Beat out as for escalopes. Place a piece of risotto filling on each. Roll up the escalopes and tie with string or secure with an orange stick. Fry in the oil. Remove and set aside. Brown the onion in the oil. Add the flour. Stir in stock and tomatoes. Bring to boil, and season. Pack the turkey breasts in an ovenware dish just large enough to hold them in a single layer. Pour the sauce over. Cook in moderate oven for 30–35 mins.

Risotto Filling

> ½ cup rice
> ½ Tbsp margarine
> 1 Tbsp chopped apricot *or* apple *or* almonds *or* chestnuts
> ½ tsp oregano *or* basil
> 1 small onion
> 1 cup stock

To make a small risotto filling, follow instructions on p. 90 for *Risotto*, using rice, chopped apricots or apples or almonds or chestnuts, and ½ tsp oregano or basil. Left-over risotto from another dish would also be quite suitable for this purpose.

Sauté Turkey

Cut fillets of turkey breast into oyster-sized pieces, and sauté as for Chicken (p. 92). (Especially good are the Almonds and the Apricots recipes.)

Turkey Legs

These can be skinned, chopped into suitably-sized pieces, and used in any stewed chicken recipe, such as Casserole, Curry, Fricassée, Stoved, etc (pp. 85–93). Try them in Irish Stew (p. 107) or Lancashire Hotpot (p. 108), instead of lamb.

Turkey Goulash with Dumplings   *Serves 4*

1½ lb turkey thighs skinned, boned, and cut into 1-inch cubes
2 Tbsp oil
1 large chopped onion
1 crushed clove of garlic
1 Tbsp flour
½ Tbsp paprika
1 Tbsp tomato purée *or* 1 small tin tomatoes
½ pt stock
salt
pinch chilli powder (optional)

Brown the turkey in the oil. Add the onion and garlic, and sweat until transparent. Stir in the flour and paprika. Mix in tomato purée and stock. Stir out lumps. Season with salt and chilli powder (optional). Bring to boil. Balance liquid with a little water or stock, and simmer till the turkey is tender.

Potato Dumplings

1 medium potato boiled and mashed
4 Tbsp S.R. flour
1 oz margarine
½ tsp mixed herbs
½ tsp salt

Rub the margarine through the flour. Add the herbs and salt. Mix into the mashed potato with enough water to form a not too stiff dough. Form into 1-inch balls. Drop into the Goulash, and simmer for 10 mins.

Turkey Burgers

Proceed exactly as for Chicken Burgers (p. 85).

Assorted Meats

Rabbit

Rabbit is an excellent white meat for the diet. Rabbit can be treated in similar ways to chicken: the legs of young ones can be sautéed (p. 92) and larger and older rabbits stewed or casseroled (p. 85).

If you find the small bones off-putting, bone the meat and cut it into 1-inch pieces. Rabbit legs can be boned and fried as in recipes given under Chicken (p. 84). They may also be boned and hammered out to make escalopes, and served as for turkey (p. 98).

Sweetbreads

Sweetbreads should be soaked in cold water for at least 20 mins, to remove blood. Blanch them – i.e. bring quickly to the boil and wash off in cold water. Pick off all fat and tough membrane.

Creamed Sweetbreads   *Serves 2*

    12 oz sweetbreads
    1 chopped onion
    1 bay leaf
    water to cover
    roux (p. 27)
    ¼ cup soya milk
    salt

Cook the sweetbreads with the onion, roughly chopped, and bay leaf in just enough water to cover. (A little white wine can replace some of the water if desired.) Season with salt. Drain off the stock. Make a Velouté (p. 34) with the stock and a roux. Whiten with the soya milk.

Cut the sweetbreads into smaller pieces and mix into the sauce.

Braised Sweetbreads   *Serves 2*

12 oz sweetbreads
2 Tbsp oil
1 sliced carrot
1 chopped onion
1½ Tbsp flour
1 tsp mixed herbs
stock as required
1 Tbsp sherry (optional)
salt, pepper

Fry the sweetbreads in the oil. Remove and set aside. Rough-chop the carrot and onion, and fry in the oil with the flour until the flour begins to brown. Add the herbs. Lay the sweetbreads on top of the vegetables and add enough stock to not quite cover the sweetbreads. Season to taste. Bring to boil, then bake uncovered in moderate oven. Baste occasionally until the sweetbreads are brown and the liquid is reduced to about half its original quantity. A Tbsp of sherry may be added with the stock if preferred.

Sweetbread Vol-au-Vents

Prepare Creamed Sweetbreads as above, adding a few button mushrooms, and cutting sweetbread into smaller pieces. Spoon into vol-au-vent cases (p. 96).

Sweetbread Escalopes

Slice cooked sweetbreads into ¼-inch thick slices. Batter and breadcrumb. Fry in deep fat until golden brown.
     Serve with Tomato Sauce (p. 33).

Veal

Veal contains very little fat, and can be braised or roasted. Because it contains so little fat it can be roasted with stuffing such as Risotto Filling (p. 99).
     Other methods of using veal are as follows.

Veal Escalopes

Slices from the hindquarters are hammered out to ¼-inch thickness, then battered and breadcrumbed. These may be treated the same ways as Fillets of Turkey Breast (p. 98).

Veal Fricassée   *Serves 4*

> 1 lb veal
> 1 chopped onion
> 1 bay leaf
> salt, pepper
> water to cover
> 2 oz margarine
> 2 oz flour
> soya milk to make up to 1 pt
> chopped parsley

Cut the veal into 1-inch cubes. Blanch, and wash in cold water to remove all scum. Return to the pan with chopped onion and bay leaf. Just cover with water. Season and simmer till tender. Melt the margarine in another pan. Mix in the flour. Stir in about ¾ pt of the broth from veal. Simmer for a few minutes to cook the roux. Add veal.

Add ¼ pt soya milk to whiten the fricassée, and balance the liquid. Do not further boil or the soya milk may curdle. Stir in a little chopped parsley, and serve.

Lunch and Supper Dishes

Shepherd's Pie   *Serves 2–3*

    8 oz minced chicken *or* turkey
    1 large onion
    1 clove garlic
    1 Tbsp oil
    ½ Tbsp flour
    1 Tbsp tomato purée
    ½ pt stock
    1 lb peeled potatoes
    1 oz margarine
    1 Tbsp soya milk (approx.)
    salt, pepper

Chop the onion and garlic, and fry them in the oil. Add the minced chicken or turkey, and brown. Add the flour, tomato purée, and stock. Season. Simmer for a few minutes. Turn into a pie-dish, and allow to cool. Boil potatoes separately, and mash with the margarine and soften with soya milk. Cover mince with the mashed potato, brush with melted margarine, and brown in a hot oven.

Moussaka   *Serves 4*

    1 lb veal
    2 Tbsp oil
    1 aubergine
    2 courgettes
    1 onion
    salt, pepper
    3–4 tomatoes
    ½ lb white cabbage
    1 clove garlic
    ½ pt stock *or* water

Cut the meat into 1-inch cubes. Slice all the vegetables. Chop the garlic. Brown the meat in the oil, in a heavy casserole. Remove the meat and the oil. Layer the vegetables and the meat back into the casserole, starting with the aubergine. Sprinkle each layer with salt and freshly ground pepper. When all the other ingredients are in the casserole, add stock or water. Pour on the oil. Bring to a simmer on top of the stove, then cook in a moderate oven for 1–1½ hrs.

Serve in the cooking dish.

Note: Any variation of vegetables can be used, including potatoes, but these should always include aubergine or courgette, tomatoes and onion. Vegetables should amount to at least two-thirds of the total volume.

A popular method of preparing this dish is to put the meat through a mincer, or finely chop. Mix it with finely chopped potato and layer this mixture with the vegetables. Moussaka can also be prepared with turkey legs or chicken thighs.

Squab Pie   *Serves 2*

Squabs are really baby crows and pigeons. When cartridges were cheap, the young birds were blasted out of their nests with shotguns and made into pies. Somehow or other, young crows became translated into cold mutton, and cooked with potatoes, apples and onions; and this is what is nowadays known as squab pie. A flavoursome version of this dish can be made by using cold chicken or turkey; and these, of course, are suitable for the diet.

> ½ lb (approx.) cooked chicken *or* turkey
> 3 apples
> 4–5 potatoes
> 3 onions
> ½ pt stock
> 1 oz (approx.) margarine
> oregano *or* thyme
> salt, pepper

Slice the apples, potatoes, onions, and cooked meat. Layer them into a margarined pie-dish, sprinkling each layer with salt and pepper and herbs. Start and finish with a layer of potatoes. Pour in the stock, and dab with margarine. Bake in a moderate oven for 45 mins, or until the potatoes are cooked through.

Chicken with Chilli

Serves 4

Our diet substitute for Chilli con Carne.

> 1 lb skinned chicken thighs
> 8 oz red kidney beans
> 2 Tbsp oil
> ¼ tsp cumin seed
> 2 chopped onions
> 1 Tbsp flour
> ½ pt any stock
> ½ tsp chilli powder
> 1 small tin tomatoes
> 1 Tbsp tomato purée
> salt

Soak beans overnight, and cook. Flour the chicken and fry in the oil. Remove and set aside. Fry the cumin seed in the oil for a second or so, add the onions, and sweat a little. Stir in the flour. Mix in the stock and the other ingredients. Add the chicken. Bring to boil. Balance liquid with a little more stock if required. Cook till chicken is tender. Mix in the cooked red beans. Re-heat thoroughly. Serve with plain boiled rice. The above will also make a substantial dish without the chicken.

Irish Stew

Serves 4 generously

> 1½ lb skinned chicken *or* turkey joints
> 2 large onions
> 2 carrots
> 1½ lb potatoes
> 1 leek *or* a few spring onions
> 2 Tbsp oil *or* margarine
> approx. 1 pt any stock
> salt, pepper

Chop the onions, carrots, and leek. Cut the potatoes into quarters. Mix half the potatoes with the other vegetables, and lay on the bottom of the pot. Lay on the chicken joints. Season with salt and pepper. Add the other half of the potatoes. Add oil or margarine. Pour over the stock. Cover and simmer gently for about 1 hr until all are tender.

Lancashire Hotpot

Serves 4

> 1½ lb skinned chicken *or* turkey joints
> 4 lamb kidneys
> 1½ lb potatoes
> 2 large onions
> ½ pt any stock
> salt, pepper
> 2 Tbsp oil

Cut the kidneys in half, and remove fat and all white tissue. Slice the potatoes and onions into ¼-inch-thick slices. Put a good layer of potatoes and onions in the bottom of an ovenware dish. Lay on the chicken joints, and kidney. Add the rest of the onions, and finish with a layer of potatoes with slices neatly overlapping. Season the stock, and pour over. Pour over the oil and cook, covered, in a moderate oven for 1½ hrs. Remove cover, and cook for further ½ hr to brown the potatoes.

Cornish Pasty

Makes 4 pasties

A *real* Cornish pasty is a two-course meal, with the meat course at one end and the sweet course at the other. The pasty is filled with beef, potato and turnip, divided by a flap of pastry from cooking apple. What is usually served, however, is a pasty stuffed with a beef, potato, and onion mixture, sometimes with added carrot or turnip. We substitute the beef with chicken, turkey, or veal.

> *Short Crust Pastry*
> 1 lb self-raising flour
> 6 oz margarine
> 3 Tbsp water
> a pinch of salt
> beaten egg white *or* soya milk
> *Filling*
> ½ lb finely chopped raw chicken, turkey, *or* veal
> 1 onion
> 2 small potatoes
> 1 small carrot
> salt, pepper

Rub the margarine through the flour till it resembles breadcrumbs. Mix in water and salt to make a fairly firm dough. Cut into 4 pieces, and roll out to 5-inch rounds.

Finely chop the vegetables and mix in chicken, turkey, or veal. Season the mixture, moisten with just a tsp of water, and place in centre of the pastry rounds. Bring up the two sides of the pastry and seal together to form a ridge on top. Brush with beaten white of egg, or soya milk, and cook for 25 mins in a hot oven.

Chicken Liver and Mushroom Pasty   *Filling for 4 pasties*

> 6 oz chicken liver
> 2 oz mushrooms
> 1 small potato
> pastry (see above)
> 1 onion
> 1 oz margarine
> salt, pepper

Cut the chicken livers into 4. Slice the mushrooms. Finely chop the onion and potato. Fry all in the margarine. Season, and fill into pastry rounds as for Cornish pasties. Cook for 25 mins in a hot oven.

Forfar Bridies   *Makes 6*

Forfar Bridies are generally made with puff pastry, but can be made with shortcrust (pp. 148–9). The filling for Forfar Bridies should be finely chopped beef and onion; but for this, we can quite well substitute chicken, turkey, or veal.

> ½ lb finely chopped (not minced) veal, turkey *or* chicken
> 1 finely chopped onion
> salt, pepper
> ½ Tbsp water
> 6 × 4 inch rounds shortcrust or puff pastry
> beaten egg white *or* Soya milk

Finely chop the meat and mix with finely chopped onion. Season, and moisten with a very little water. Put the filling to one side of the centre of the pastry round, and fold "turnover" style. Brush edges of pastry with water, and seal. Glaze with white of egg, or soya milk. Cook in a hot oven for 25 mins.

Savoury Pancakes

Serves 4

Using whole eggs, the usual recipe for basic batter includes 4 oz flour to ¼ pt milk, plus 1 or 2 eggs. As we shall only be using egg whites, we must increase the flour content as follows.

> 5 oz plain flour
> 2 egg whites
> ½ pt soya milk
> a pinch of salt
> 1 Tbsp oil

Mix the egg whites into the milk. Add the flour and salt, and beat to a smooth cream. Allow the batter to stand for about 1 hour. It will thicken slightly.

Brush a hot omelette pan with oil and pour in about 2 Tbsp batter. Swirl the pan to spread the batter evenly. Cook to golden brown. Turn with a spatula, and cook other side. Leave tossing the pancake to show-off cooks. To do this successfully calls for some expertise, and a pan which – because it is kept solely for pancakes – does not stick.

Pancakes may be prepared hours before required. Just stack them interleaved with greaseproof paper.

The list of fillings need be limited only by your imagination or by what is available. Here are only a few suggestions.

Mushroom and Onion Filling

Sweat chopped onions in margarine for 1 min, then add sliced mushrooms and cook till the mushrooms are shiny. Moisten with White Sauce (p. 30), or add some soya milk or stock thickened with cornflour. Season to taste.

Curry Filling

Use left-overs of curried chicken. If this includes some left-over rice, heat the rice separately. It is difficult to reheat thoroughly any very thick mixture. Serve with a spoonful of chutney on each pancake.

Tuna and Pepper (Pimento) Filling

Chop a small onion and sweat in oil drained from a tin of tuna. Shred the peppers, and sweat with the onion for another minute or so. Flake the tuna, and mix into the pepper and onion. Season to taste.

Sliced mushrooms may be substituted for the shredded peppers.

Smoked Haddock Filling

Prepare as for Fish Savoury (p. 79). Any of the other fish given in that recipe can also be used.

Paella   *Serves 2–3*

The traditional recipe calls for pork and *chorizo* (Spain's highly spiced sausage) and saffron. It also calls for seafood such as lobster, crayfish, clams, and mussels. We cannot use the pork and the *chorizo* in our diet. Seafood and saffron are expensive and can be difficult to find; but we can find substitutes for these and still produce a fine-flavoured dish. The pundits say that turmeric, for example, should not be used in place of saffron, but on several occasions in Spain I have come across excellent Paella which most certainly contained turmeric.

The name "paella" derives from "paelleria", the pan that Spaniards use for cooking this dish. In its absence, use a large casserole. The following is an inexpensive version of Paella which calls for the minimum of preparation.

> 4–5 oz cooked chicken
> 1 tin tuna fish
> 1 large onion
> 1 clove garlic
> 2 or 3 tomatoes, tinned or fresh
> 1 small red or green pepper (or both)
> 1 Tbsp oil
> 2 oz green peas
> 1 cup long-grain rice
> 3 cups chicken stock
> ½ tsp oregano
> ½ tsp turmeric
> salt, pepper

Note: the three-to-one ratio of stock to rice must be adhered to. The quantities of the other ingredients can vary according to availability and taste.

Chop the onion and garlic. Rough-chop the tomatoes and

peppers. Cut the chicken into 1-inch chunks. Flake the tuna. Fry the onion and garlic in the oil. Add the rice, and thoroughly coat the grains with oil. Add the stock, and all other ingredients. Bring to the boil, cover, and finish cooking in a moderately hot oven for 20 mins, or until the rice is tender, and has absorbed all the stock.

Macaroni with Mushroom Sauce   *Serves 4*

8–12 oz macaroni
6–8 oz mushrooms
2½ oz margarine
1 pt Velouté Sauce (p. 34)
salt
pepper

Cook the macaroni in boiling salted water until they are *al dente* i.e. just tender. *Al dente* literally means "to the teeth", suggesting "with a bite to it".

Drain macaroni and toss in ½ oz of the margarine. While the macaroni is cooking, slice and sauté the mushrooms in the remaining margarine, boil velouté and mix in mushrooms. Check seasoning.

Serve macaroni with the sauce poured over.

Pasta Shells with Smoked Fish   *Serves 4*

All pasta is made from the same basic recipe; but somehow or other, altering the shape of the pasta seems also to alter the flavour. Some shapes seem to go better with certain ingredients than with others. This recipe and the one below go well with pasta shells.

8 oz pasta shells
1 lb smoked haddock
1 pt mixed soya milk and water *or* water only
1 onion
2 oz flour
2½ oz margarine
freshly ground pepper
salt

Cook the pasta shells in boiling salted water *al dente*. Drain and toss in ½ oz margarine.

Meanwhile, poach the fish in the milk and water. Drain, and save liquid. Chop the onion, and sweat in the margarine. Mix in flour, add liquid from fish, stir out lumps. Season with pepper (there should be enough salt from the fish), bring to boil, and simmer for a few minutes. Remove skin from fish. Break the fish, and add to sauce. Mix the sauce through the hot cooked pasta shells.

Pasta Shells with Chicken

Simply mix a Chicken Fricassée (p. 89) into the cooked pasta shells. Serve with a sprinkling of chopped parsley.

Spaghetti and Tomato   *Serves 4*

> 8–12 oz spaghetti
> 1 onion
> 1 clove garlic
> 1½ oz margarine
> 1 tin tomatoes
> 1 tsp oregano
> salt
> freshly ground black pepper

Boil the spaghetti in boiling salted water. Drain and toss in ½ oz of the margarine. While the spaghetti is boiling, slice the onion, crush the garlic and sauté in the remaining margarine. Add tomatoes, and oregano. Boil to pulp. Season with salt and freshly ground pepper. Ladle over the spaghetti.

Spaghetti Tetrazzini   *Serves 4*

> 8 oz spaghetti
> 2½ oz margarine
> 2 onions
> 8 oz mushrooms
> 8 oz cooked chicken

1 pt chicken Velouté (p. 34)
1 Tbsp lemon juice
salt
freshly ground black pepper

Cook spaghetti in boiling salted water. Drain and toss in ½ oz margarine. While spaghetti is cooking, slice the onions and mushrooms. Shred the cooked chicken. Sweat the onion in the margarine. Add the mushrooms, and cook till shiny. Add the chicken Velouté, lemon juice, and shredded chicken. Season with salt and freshly ground pepper. Ladle over the hot cooked spaghetti.

Spaghetti with Chicken Livers   *Serves 4*

8 oz spaghetti
1 lb chicken livers
1 large onion
4 oz mushrooms
2½ Tbsp oil
1 tsp oregano
1 Tbsp flour
2 cups stock
salt
freshly ground black pepper

Cut the chicken livers in two. Slice the onion and mushrooms, and sweat in the oil. Add the chicken livers and oregano. Stir in flour and cook until ingredients start to brown. Add the tomatoes, and stock. Season with salt and freshly-ground pepper. Simmer for about 15 mins.

Serve livers ladled over the hot cooked spaghetti.

Pizza

Shop-bought pizzas are hopelessly unsuitable for this diet because, apart from forbidden natural ingredients such as butter and cheese, some of them contain additives which are better avoided. The proper dough for pizza is leavened with yeast, which means that the making of it requires forward planning and time-consuming preparation. Here is a quick, easy alternative.

Quick Pizza Paste   *Serves 2*

> 6 oz self-raising flour
> 1 oz margarine
> ½ tsp salt
> 1 tsp mixed herbs

Mix flour, herbs, and salt. Rub in the margarine. Mix in enough water to make a soft dough. Cut in two and pin out to two round shapes. Place on oven tray or use them to line flan rings.

Pizza Filling   *Serves 2*

> 1 clove garlic
> 1 small onion
> 2 oz mushrooms
> 1 oz margarine
> salt, pepper
> 1 Tbsp tomato purée
> 4 sliced tomatoes
> 1 small green pepper
> 1 tin anchovies

Crush the garlic, slice onion and mushrooms, and sweat in the margarine. Season. Spread the tomato purée over the pizza dough. Sprinkle the mushrooms and onion over. Arrange the sliced tomatoes in place over the onion and mushrooms. Shred the green pepper, and scatter on. Criss-cross the anchovies over all. Cook in a hot oven for 15–20 mins.

Tomato purée is, of course, a necessary part of the pizza, but the mushroom and onion filling can be replaced by other ingredients, the choice of which need be limited only by your imagination. Try, for instance, tinned tuna mixed with a little tomato ketchup, chopped cooked chicken moistened with a little Brown Sauce (p. 31), or chopped chicken livers moistened with Devilled Sauce (p. 94); but always finish with the shredded peppers and the anchovies – unless, of course, you don't like anchovies!

Some Vegetable Dishes

Home-Baked Beans   *Serves 2–3*

> ½ lb haricot or butter beans
> 1 chopped onion
> 1 oz margarine
> water to cover
> 1 Tbsp syrup
> ½ pt tomato juice
> salt, pepper

Soak the beans overnight. Wash beans and place in a casserole with the chopped onion, margarine, syrup and tomato juice. Add water to just cover the beans. Season, cover tightly, and cook in a moderate oven till tender – at least 4 hrs.

Baked Beans – Tinned

The better brands contain no additives and so they are perfectly safe for our diet.

Curried Beans   *Serves 4*

> ½ lb dried beans (any type)
> 1 carrot
> equal turnip
> 1 onion
> 1 cooking apple
> 1 Tbsp des. coconut
> ½ Tbsp curry powder
> 2 Tbsp oil
> 1 Tbsp flour
> 1 Tbsp chutney
> 1 Tbsp lemon juice
> ½ Tbsp tomato purée
> ½ pt any stock
> salt

Soak and cook the beans. Chop the vegetables and apple, and sweat in the oil with the curry powder for 2–3 mins. Stir in the

flour. Add all other ingredients, and cook until vegetables are
tender. Mix in the cooked beans, and simmer for about 15 mins.
    Serve with boiled rice.

Bean Goulash   *Serves 4*

> ½ lb cooked dried beans (any type)
> 1 large onion
> 1 carrot
> equal turnip
> ½ red pepper
> ½ green pepper
> 1 clove garlic
> 2 Tbsp oil
> 1 Tbsp flour
> 1 Tbsp paprika
> pinch chilli powder *or* Cayenne
> 1 small tin tomatoes
> ½ pt any stock
> salt

Cut the vegetables into ½-inch dice. Sweat in the oil with the
crushed garlic for 2–3 mins. Add the flour and the paprika. Stir in
the tomatoes and the stock. Add the chilli or cayenne, and salt to
taste. Cook until vegetables are tender. Add the beans, and
simmer for about 15 mins.
    Serve with boiled rice, or pasta.
    A can of baked beans can be substituted for the dried beans.

Bubble and Squeak

Chop together approximately equal quantities of cold cooked
potatoes and cabbage. Season with salt and pepper and fry in
margarine. (About 2 oz margarine per lb of vegetables.) Keep
turning in the pan until margarine is mixed through, then brown
on both sides.

Colcannon

Some cookery books give exactly the same recipe for this dish as
for Bubble and Squeak, but I think this is completely wrong.

Colcannon can be prepared with re-heated cooked vegetables, but should properly be prepared from vegetables cooked freshly for the purpose.

Simply mash together approximately equal quantities of cooked potato, carrot, turnip, and cabbage. Mix in some margarine. Season with salt and pepper, and serve.

Clapshot

A near-relation of Colcannon, from the Orkney Islands. Cook together equal quantities of swede and potatoes. (The flavour is vastly superior to that of the same mixture cooked separately.) Drain and mash. Season with salt and plenty of freshly ground pepper.

Champ

A similar dish from Ireland. Raw spring onions, including the green part, are chopped fairly finely and mixed into mashed potato.

Cauliflower Fritters

Cook cauliflower florets until just tender. Drain and allow to cool. Make a batter with self-raising flour and water mixed to the consistency of double cream. Season with salt. Dip florets in batter, and shake off surplus. Fry in deep hot oil until crisp. Drain on kitchen paper. Serve with Tomato Sauce (p. 33).

Mushroom Fritters

Proceed as for Cauliflower Fritters, but use raw mushrooms.

Mushrooms on Toast

Allow 2 oz plus of mushrooms per person. Slice the mushrooms. Fry in margarine until mushrooms are shiny. Season with salt and freshly-ground pepper. Pile on hot toast and serve immediately.

Field mushrooms and other wild fungi have a flavour much superior to that of the cultivated variety, but they also have a much higher water content. Cooked in the margarine, they will exude a considerable quantity of liquid. When they are shiny, remove them from the pan with a perforated spoon. Reduce the liquid until only about 1 Tbsp remains, then return mushrooms to pan and re-heat in the reduced liquid.

Rice and Mushroom Patties

Serves 2–3

1 cup rice
¼ lb sliced mushrooms
1 oz margarine
3 cups stock
1 sliced onion
salt, pepper
batter (p. 60)
breadcrumbs
oil for frying
Tomato Sauce (p. 33)

Follow the instructions on p. 95 for Risotto. When the risotto is cooked, stir so as to break up the rice deliberately. This will help to bind the mixture. Put aside and allow to cool. When quite cold, shape into 4 or 6 round, flat cakes. Coat with batter, then breadcrumbs. Fry in hot oil.

Serve with Tomato Sauce.

Baked Potatoes

With Mushrooms

Serves 4

4 large potatoes
4 oz mushrooms
1 onion
1 clove garlic, chopped
1 oz margarine
½ cup soya milk
salt, pepper

Bake the potatoes in a hot oven for approximately 1¼–1½ hrs.

Chop the onion, slice the mushrooms. Sweat the onion and garlic in the margarine until transparent. Add the mushrooms, and cook till mushrooms are shiny. Cut the potatoes in half, longways. Scoop out flesh. Roughly mash, and mix with the milk. Season. Mix in the mushrooms and onions. Pile back into the potato shells, and brown under the grill.

With Tomatoes and Anchovy   *Serves 4*

> 4 large potatoes
> 1 small tin tomatoes
> 1 tin anchovies
> 1 onion
> 1 clove garlic
> 1 oz margarine
> Cayenne pepper
> salt

Bake the potatoes in a hot oven for approx. 1¼–1½ hrs. Drain and roughly chop the tomatoes. Drain the anchovies (saving the oil) and chop. Chop the onion and garlic. Sweat the onion and garlic in the margarine and the oil drained from the anchovies. Mix in the tomatoes and anchovies. Add a pinch of Cayenne pepper. Cut the potatoes in half, longways. Scoop out flesh, roughly mash, and mix with the tomato and anchovy mixture. Pile back into potato shells and brown under the grill.

With Smoked Fish   *Serves 4*

> 4 large potatoes
> 4 oz smoked haddock
> 1 onion
> 1 oz margarine
> ½ cup soya milk
> cayenne pepper
> chopped parsley
> salt if required

Bake the potatoes in a hot oven for approx. 1¼–1½ hrs. Poach the fish in the milk. Chop the onion, and sweat in the margarine. Cut potatoes in half, longways. Scoop out flesh, and roughly mash. Break the fish and fold into the mashed potato along with the milk, onion, and pepper. Check if any salt is needed (the fish is salty). Pile back into potato shells, and serve with a sprinkling of chopped parsley.

Stovies (Stewed Potatoes)   *Serves 2*

> 7–8 good sized potatoes
> 3–4 onions
> 2 oz margarine
> salt, pepper
> bare ½ pt stock
> chicken meat scraps (optional)

Cut potatoes and onions in ½-in thick slices. Sweat in the margarine. Season with salt and pepper, and add the stock. Cover closely and simmer gently for 1½ hrs. Shake occasionally to prevent sticking. Scraps of cooked white meat, such as chicken, can be added.

Serve in deep plates, with bread.

Potato and Bean Cutlets   *Makes 4*

> ½ lb boiled and mashed potatoes
> breadcrumbs
> 1 tin baked beans
> batter (p. 60)
> oil for frying
> Tomato Sauce (p. 33)

Drain the beans and mix well into the hot mashed potatoes, but do not break the beans too much. Shape the mixture into cutlets. Allow to cool thoroughly. Coat with batter and breadcrumbs. Fry in either shallow or deep oil.

Serve with Tomato Sauce.

Ratatouille   *Serves 2 for main dish*

> 4 courgettes
> 1 clove garlic
> 2 onions
> 1 red pepper

1 green pepper
2 Tbsp oil
1 small tin tomatoes
salt, pepper

Crush the garlic, and thickly slice (about ¼-inch thick) the courgettes, onions, and peppers. Sweat all in the oil. Add the tomatoes. Season lightly. Simmer with a lid on, until tender (25–30 mins). Shake occasionally to avoid burning, and check liquid level, adding a little water if necessary.

May be served simply as a vegetable accompaniment, or as a main dish dressed on a risotto of rice, or on macaroni.

To serve as a salad, cool, and stir in 1 Tbsp lemon juice or vinegar and 1 Tbsp oil.

Vegetable Pie

Almost any mixture of cooked vegetables can be used for a pie, but should include at least one pulse – such as beans or peas – to add protein. The moistening sauce can be either White (p. 30) – as for Fricassée – or, if you are going to use tomatoes, Brown Sauce (p. 31). Fresh vegetables are preferable but tinned vegetables are acceptable provided they are free of artificial additives.

Method 1 with White Sauce   *Serves 4*

1 raw onion
2 oz raw mushrooms
4 oz cooked peas *or* sliced green beans
4 oz cooked sliced carrot
4 oz cooked butter beans
2 oz margarine
1 oz flour
½ pt stock *or* cooking liquid from the vegetables
salt, pepper
shortcrust pastry (p. 149)

Slice the onion and mushrooms and sweat them in the margarine. Mix in the flour. Add the stock, hot but not boiling, stirring to avoid lumps. Bring to boil. Mix in the cooked vegetables. Turn into a pie-dish and cover with short pastry. Bake in a moderate oven for about 20 mins.

Method 2 with Brown Sauce
Serves 4

> 1 sliced raw onion
> 1 crushed clove garlic
> 2 oz sliced mushrooms
> 1 small tin tomatoes
> 1 small tin baked beans
> 4 oz cooked carrots
> 4 oz cooked peas
> 1 Tbsp flour
> 2 Tbsp oil
> ½ cup stock (approx.)
> salt, pepper
> shortcrust pastry (p. 149)

Brown the flour in the oil but do not allow to burn. Mix in the onion, garlic and mushrooms. Add the tinned tomatoes and the ½ cup of stock or cooking liquor from the vegetables to make a heavy sauce. (The exact amount will depend on the amount of liquid in the tomatoes.) Add the cooked vegetables. Bring to boil. Turn into a pie-dish. Allow to cool. Cover with short pastry. Cook in a moderate oven for about 20 mins.

The pie may also be covered with mashed potatoes, Shepherd's Pie style. For a top and bottom pastry version, double the amount of pastry and halve the quantity of vegetables.

Salads

The salad is the most versatile dish on the menu. It can be served as a starter, as the accompaniment to a main dish, or as a main dish in itself. In effect, it is the simplest way of adding variety to a meal; but additionally with a little imagination and care for the choice and arrangement of the ingredients, salad can dress the table in a way that will provide the all-important eye appeal which stimulates appetite.

I have listed here only some of the many possibilities for a salad dish; but keep in mind that practically any savoury ingredient can be mixed with any kind of fruit or vegetable, and it will be realised that the possible combinations of texture and flavour cover a range that is almost infinite. You will find it interesting, also, to serve two or three mixtures side by side on the one dish – or to mix several together. For decorative effect, try using the eye-catching green of sliced Chinese gooseberries (kiwi fruit), or the black of pickled walnuts. Additional colour is achieved by leaving the skin on apples, pears, and cucumbers; and the skin, of course, also adds variety to the texture of the whole.

Olive oil is the classic salad oil but many prefer a blander flavoured oil. Any of the popular vegetable cooking oils such as sunflower or corn oil will serve. Olive oil is also expensive, but it can be mixed in any proportion with the various vegetable oils to add a little flavour.

Remember, finally, that quantities of the various ingredients are unimportant – and so give free rein to your fancy!

Apple, Potato and Caper

Diced, cooked potato with diced, whole raw apple. Moisten with Soya Mayonnaise (p. 35). Dress on lettuce leaf. Sprinkle with capers.

Apple, Orange, and Pear

Slice apples, pears, and oranges. Moisten with Vinaigrette (p. 38) to which a little mustard has been added.

Apple and Shrimp

Dice the apples. Mix with the shrimps. Moisten with Soya Mayonnaise (p. 35).

Apricot and Pepper

Slice tinned apricot caps, and mix with chopped red and green peppers. Moisten with juice from the apricots. Season with just a touch of salt.

Asparagus and Chicken

Dress asparagus tips on little slices of cold cooked chicken. Sprinkle with chopped walnuts. Moisten with Vinaigrette (p. 38).

Banana, Tomato and Tangerine

Mix sliced tomatoes and bananas with lemon juice. Serve dressed round a heap of tangerine segments.

Beetroot

Cut small pickled beetroots in slices, or large beets in dice. Sprinkle with finely-chopped onion and parsley. Dribble a little salad oil over.

Celery and Apple

Chop celery in segments across the stalk. Mix with sliced

apple. Moisten with a little soya milk and lemon juice. Season with salt and white pepper.

Chicory and Celery

Slice chicory and celery. Mix in some roughly-chopped gherkin and a few black olives. Dress on lettuce or curly endive – preferably the latter. Moisten with Vinaigrette (p. 38).

Coleslaw

Strictly speaking, Coleslaw is finely-shredded white cabbage moistened with vinaigrette. The cabbage, however, is often mixed with finely-shredded celery, or carrots, or grated apple, or with a combination of all three.

Cucumber and Apple

Chop cucumber and apple into ½-inch dice. Season with salt. Moisten with lemon juice and a little soya milk.

Cucumber, Tomato and French Beans

Cut all in small dice. Moisten with Vinaigrette (p. 38). French beans, if tender and fresh, can be used raw; otherwise, use cooked beans.

Endive and Avocado

Cut the flesh of the avocado in slices, and dress on curly endive. Sprinkle with chopped nuts. Dress lightly with lemon juice and salad oil.

Florida Salad

Mix chopped pineapple, banana and apple with grapefruit segments. Moisten with Soya Mayonnaise (p. 35). Dress on shredded lettuce.

Grapefruit and Orange

Dress small segments of orange and grapefruit on shredded lettuce. Strew with a few grapes and hazelnuts. Moisten with Vinaigrette (p. 38).

Herring Salad

Cut pickled herrings into strips, and mix with diced cooked potato and sliced raw apple. Moisten with Vinaigrette (p. 38). Garnish with shredded gherkins.

Kipper Salad

Raw kipper fillets cut in strips and mixed with a little chopped onion. Moisten with Vinaigrette (p. 38).

Mushroom and Carrot

Cook the carrot (but leave with a "bite") and cut into strips. Mix with sliced raw button mushrooms. Add a few green peas and/or some finely-shredded green pepper. Dress with Vinaigrette (p. 38).

Salade Niçoise

> French beans (cooked)
> potatoes (cold cooked)
> tomatoes
> tinned anchovies
> Vinaigrette (p. 38)
> a few capers

Quantities are not critical, but French beans should be the dominant ingredient. Cut the French beans lengthwise into fine strips. Cut the potatoes and tomatoes into small slices. Shred the anchovies. Mix all with the vinaigrette. Sprinkle with a few capers.

Peach and Pepper

Tinned sliced peaches mixed with strips of red and green pepper. Dress with lemon juice and a pinch of salt. Leave a little syrup clinging to the peaches.

Potato Salad

Cooked diced potato mixed with finely-chopped onion. Moisten with lemon juice and a little soya milk. Season with salt and pepper. Sprinkle with chopped parsley.

If new potatoes are used, these should be sliced rather than diced, mixed with finely-chopped spring onions, and moistened with Soya Mayonnaise (p. 38).

Red Cabbage

Drain pickled cabbage, and mix in a little salad oil. Serve on lettuce leaves. Sprinkle with chopped parsley. May also be mixed with sliced raw onion.

Red Kidney Beans

Mix cooked kidney beans with chopped raw onion. Moisten with Vinaigrette (p. 38) to which a pinch of chilli powder has been added.

Rice and Mushroom

Mix finely-sliced raw button mushrooms and a few green peas with plain boiled rice. Moisten with Vinaigrette (p. 38).

Rice and Peppers

Mix plain boiled rice with diced red and green peppers. Moisten with Vinaigrette (p. 38).

Russian Salad

Cut carrot and turnip into short strips (rather than dice). Cook, leaving a "bite". Mix with cooked, short-cut French beans, and cooked fresh or frozen peas. Moisten with Soya Mayonnaise (p. 35).

Originally, Russian Salad had anchovy, gherkins, and capers mixed through, but this is no longer the case.

Salade Polonaise

Add strips of pickled herring, and gherkins, to Russian Salad.

Sardine Salad

Dress tinned sardines on lettuce. Strew with chopped chives and parsley. Moisten with lemon juice and oil from the tin.

Tabbouleh (a salad from the Middle East)

        2 oz chopped mint
        2 oz spring onion
        8 oz cooked *burghul or* cooked cracked wheat
        4 Tbsp salad oil
        salt, pepper
        4 oz chopped parsley
        4 oz chopped tomato
        2 Tbsp lemon juice

Mix all ingredients together.

Note: *Burghul*, or the very similar Bulgarian cracked wheat is available from most health food shops.

Tomato Salad

Slice firm tomatoes and arrange on a dish. Sprinkle with salt. Strew with finely-chopped onion. Dress with lemon juice, and salad oil.

Waldorf Salad

Mix chopped apples, bananas, celery, and walnuts, with Soya Mayonnaise (p. 35). Serve on lettuce.

Sweets

Apples Baked in Wine   *Serves 4*

    4 tart apples
    4 tsp raspberry jam
    1 Tbsp caster sugar
    1 glass white wine

Core the apples – but not all the way through. Fill with raspberry jam. Pack into an ovenware dish just large enough to hold them. Sprinkle with sugar, and pour over 1 glass white wine. Cover with foil, and bake in a moderate oven until soft – approx. 40 mins.

Apple Charlotte   *Serves 4*

    1 lb cooking apples
    4 oz (approx.) margarine
    thinly sliced bread to line the dish
    1 Tbsp lemon juice
    2 Tbsp water
    3 oz sugar
    1 clove
    pinch of ground cinnamon

Generously coat a deep ovenware dish with margarine. Spread the bread with margarine. Line the dish with bread slices, margarine side in, making sure they overlap. Peel, core, and slice the apples. Stew with lemon juice, water, sugar, and a knob of margarine. Add a clove and a pinch of cinnamon. Turn into the lined dish, cover with overlapping slices of margarined bread. Bake in a moderately hot oven for 30 mins.

Free the Charlotte with a palette knife run down the side of the dish, and turn out.

Serve with custard made with soya milk (p. 38).

Apple Crumble

Serves 4

    1 lb apples
    4 oz sugar
    cinnamon
    1 Tbsp lemon juice
    2 Tbsp water
    8 oz plain flour
    4 oz margarine

Core and slice the apples, to fill a pie-dish. Add 2 oz of the sugar, a pinch of cinnamon, lemon juice, and 2 Tbsp water. Rub the remaining sugar and the margarine into the flour, until it resembles breadcrumbs. Spread over the apples, and cook in a moderately hot oven for 30 mins.

Apricots, gooseberries, plums, and rhubarb can all be used in the same way.

Baked Apple Dumplings

Peel and core apples and cut in half. Place each half on a 3-inch square of sweetcrust pastry (p. 150). Add sugar and a pinch of cinnamon. Bring up corners of pastry, and seal edges into pyramid shape. Brush lightly with water, sprinkle with granulated sugar. Bake in moderate oven for 30 mins.

Apple Fritters

Serves 4

    3–4 apples
    flour and caster sugar for coating and dredging
    Fritter batter
    4 oz plain flour
    ¼ pt tepid water
    ½ Tbsp oil
    pinch of salt
    1 egg-white

Mix flour, water, oil and salt to a smooth batter. Beat the white of egg stiffly and fold gently into batter. If possible it is better to prepare the batter an hour or so beforehand and allow it to stand.

The egg-white is beaten and folded into the batter immediately before use.

Core the apples and cut into round slices ¼-inch thick. Dip the apple slices in flour mixed with caster sugar (this helps batter to adhere), coat well with batter and cook in hot, deep oil until they brown and puff out. When they float, turn, so that both sides are equally browned. Lift out with perforated spoon and drain on kitchen paper. Dredge with caster sugar.

Serve with Apricot or Lemon Sauce (p. 39).

Apple Snow   *Serves 4*

> 4 apples
> juice of ½ lemon
> white of 2 eggs
> 4 oz sugar
> pinch salt

Peel and core apples. Cook to pulp. Mix in sugar, lemon juice, and salt. Allow to cool.

Beat egg whites stiffly. Fold into apple purée and serve in glasses.

Apple Ruin

> 1 dessert apple per person
> caster sugar
> lemon juice
> bitter chocolate

Grate the apples with their skin still on. Sprinkle with lemon juice and caster sugar. Pile grated apple in individual dishes and grate plain (bitter) chocolate over.

Serve with soya milk or non-dairy-fat "cream".

Apricot Condé   *Serves 4*

> 1 × 12 oz tin apricot halves
> ½ pkt lemon *or* orange jelly
> 1 pt rice pudding (p. 140)

Prepare a rice pudding with soya milk (p. 24). Turn into a deep serving dish, and allow to cool. Drain the syrup from 1 tin of apricot halves and lay them out over the rice. Make a lemon or orange jelly, using the syrup from the apricots to replace some of the water. When the jelly cools, pour over the apricots and allow to set.

Suitable also for peaches and pears. With pears, a red jelly is recommended.

Banana Custard
Serves 4

> 4 bananas
> 1 pt custard (p. 38)
> jam

Put a generous layer of jam in the bottom of a glass dish. Cover with a layer of sliced banana. Prepare a custard with soya milk. Pour over the bananas, and allow to cool.

This dish should not be prepared overnight, otherwise the bananas will turn black and the custard will disintegrate.

Christmas Pudding
Makes 4-pounder

> ½ lb self-raising flour
> ½ lb margarine
> ½ lb sultanas
> ¼ lb mixed peel
> 2 Tbsp black treacle
> 2 tsp mixed spice
> ½–¾ pt stout
> ½ lb breadcrumbs
> ½ lb raisins
> ½ lb currants
> ¼ lb soft brown sugar
> 2 oz ground almonds
> ½ tsp salt

Rub the margarine through the flour. Mix in all the dry ingredients. Warm the treacle to thin it, and pour over the dry ingredients. Mix in enough of the stout to make a stiff batter. Turn into a margarined basin. Cover with foil, and steam for 4 hrs.

This pudding can be stored in a cool place for a week or so. Re-heat for 4 hrs. Serve with Rum or Almond Sauce (p. 39).

Note: The above recipe makes a large pudding of over 4 lb. For a small pudding, halve the quantities. Alternatively, divide the full recipe into two basins, and hold one pudding back for New Year's Day.

Flamri (Flumry)   *Serves 4*

> ½ pt white wine
> ½ pt water
> 4 egg whites
> 3 oz sugar
> 3 oz semolina

Boil the water and wine. Stir in sugar and semolina, and cook over a low heat for about 10 mins until the mixture is thick. Cool to blood heat, and fold in the stiffly beaten white of egg. Turn the mixture into a mould which has been rinsed with cold water, and chill for about 3 hrs.

Turn out, and serve with a fruit purée, such as apricot or raspberry, spooned over the top.

Could also be prepared with ground rice in place of the semolina.

Frosted Banana Mousse   *Serves 4*

> 3 bananas
> 2 Tbsp caster sugar
> 2 stiffly beaten egg whites
> 1 Tbsp lemon juice
> 3 Tbsp orange *or* pineapple juice

Mash the bananas with the sugar and juices. Fold in the beaten egg whites. Fill into melba glasses or goblets and refrigerate.

Fruit Flan

Serves 4–6

> sweet crust pastry (p. 150)
> soft or tinned fruit
> *Glaze*
> ½ pt fruit juice
> 1 Tbsp cornflour *or* arrowroot
> 2 oz sugar
> 1 Tbsp lemon juice

Line a flan ring with sweetcrust pastry, fill with dried beans or peas to hold pastry down during cooking process, and bake in moderate oven for 15 mins. Remove peas and return to oven to brown for 5–10 mins. Allow pastry to cool. Fill with fruit such as raspberries or strawberries, or well-drained tinned fruit.

For the glaze, mix cornflour with a little water. Boil fruit juice, sugar, and lemon juice, and pour over mixed cornflour. Return to pan, and boil until clear. Colour pink with food colouring. Cool slightly. Pour over fruit in flan case. When quite cold, pipe on Decorating Cream (p. 40).

Ginger Pudding

Serves 4

> 12 oz self-raising flour
> 5 oz margarine
> soya milk
> 6 oz golden syrup
> ½ tsp ground ginger
> *Syrup sauce*
> ¼ pt syrup
> 1 Tbsp custard powder
> ¼ pt water
> pinch salt

Rub the margarine through the flour and ground ginger. Heat the syrup to thin it. Mix into the flour and margarine with enough milk to make a stiff batter. Put about 1 Tbsp of syrup into a margarined basin. Pour in the batter. Cover with foil, and steam for 2 hrs. Serve with Syrup Sauce. Boil syrup with the water and salt. Mix custard powder with a little water and pour the syrup/water over. Return to saucepan and boil for 2 mins to cook. Note that the salt *must* be used, otherwise the sauce will taste insipid.

Marmalade Pudding

Proceed as for Ginger Pudding (p. 136), but substitute marmalade for golden syrup, and omit ginger. Serve with Marmalade Sauce, which can be prepared as Jam Sauce (p. 39).

Gooseberry Fool
Serves 4

½ lb green gooseberries
2 Tbsp sugar
2 Tbsp approx. water
½ pt cold custard sauce (p. 38)

Cook gooseberries to pulp with the sugar and water. Sieve and cool. Mix with the cold custard. Serve in glasses with fingers of sweetcrust pastry (p. 150).

Lemon Meringue Pie
Serves 4

½ oz custard powder
2 Tbsp lemon juice made up with water to ¼ pt
1 oz margarine
2 oz sugar
sweet crust pastry (p. 150)
Meringue topping
2 egg whites
4 oz sugar

Prepare a flan case as for Fruit Flan (p. 136). Mix the custard powder with a little water. Boil lemon juice and water with the sugar, and pour over mixed custard powder. Return to pan, and cook until thickened and transparent. Stir in the margarine. Spread into pastry case, and allow to cool.

For the meringue topping, beat the whites stiffly. Fold in the sugar. Pile over the flan. Cook in a cool oven until meringue is set and lightly browned (approx. 1 hr). Variations on the above could be to spread the pastry case with a purée of apricots prepared from either tinned or dried apricots, or with a purée of apples to which a little lemon juice has been added.

Melon Frappé

Cut the top off a small melon, and scoop out the inside with a spoon. Remove seeds, and rough-chop the flesh. Mix with Orange Sorbet (p. 143) and 1 Tbsp of kirsch. Refill melon case.
   Serve immediately.

Orange Custard

Allow 1 orange per person. Remove the skin and pith from oranges, and cut across the segments to make ¼-inch thick slices. Proceed as for Banana Custard (p. 134), using apricot jam.

Orange Praline   *Serves 4*

   4 oz sugar
   1 Tbsp water
   4 oz chopped almonds *or* other nuts
   1 × 12 oz tin tangerines

Make a toffee by boiling the sugar and water until sugar begins to colour. Mix in the nuts, pour out on to an oiled tray, and allow to cool. When set, the toffee should be very brittle. Crush with a rolling pin or similar blunt instrument, and sprinkle over the tangerines.

Pancakes (Crêpes)

Basic batter is the same as for Savoury Pancakes (p. 110). The pancakes can be prepared in advance. They may be spread with jam or fruit purée, then rolled or folded. Alternatively, with a sprinkling of lemon juice and sugar, they can be served as Lemon Pancakes.

Crêpe Suzette
Serves 4

This is a pancake for a grand occasion.

>8 pancakes
>2 oz cube sugar
>2 oranges
>2 Tbsp Brandy
>2 oz margarine
>2 Tbsp water
>2 Tbsp Cointreau *or* Grand Marnier

Rub the cube sugar over the zest of the oranges, and place in a chafing-dish with the water. Boil till the sugar starts to brown. Add the juice of the oranges, and the margarine. Bring to boil. Add the Cointreau (or Grand Marnier), keeping the dish hot. Dip each pancake separately in the mixture, and fold into four. (This is easily done with tongs, or with spoon and fork.) Stack on one side of the chafing-dish. When all the pancakes have been dipped, tilt the pan so that the sauce runs to the side away from the pancakes. Add the brandy, bring to boil, and set alight. (Take care to hold your face well away from the dish during this operation.)

Serve the crêpes with the sauce spooned over.

An alternative method to rubbing sugar cubes over the zest of orange, is to pare the zest thinly from the orange, and then to shred finely and boil with the sugar and water.

Decked Plums
Serves 4

>1 lb fresh plums
>½ glass red wine
>1 Tbsp sugar
>*Topping*
>2 egg whites
>4 oz caster sugar

Stone the plums. Cook the halves in the sugar and wine until they are soft but not pulped. Place in shallow ovenware dish.

For the topping, beat the whites stiffly with half the sugar. Fold in the remaining sugar. Spread over the plums, and bake in a moderate oven till topping is brown.

Fresh Pineapple

Cut the top and tail off a fresh pineapple. Stand pineapple on a board and cut off skin in vertical strips. It is permissible to leave the little brown tufts which you will see when the skin is removed. Cut pineapple into round slices, and use an apple-corer to remove the hard centre from each slice. Layer the rings in a deep, narrow dish, with a generous sprinkling of caster sugar on each layer. Just moisten with 1 Tbsp of water, or kirsch. Keep in fridge for 24 hrs, turning slices occasionally. The sugar should then be completely dissolved into a light syrup.

Pineapple Meringue   Serves 4–6

Cut a fresh pineapple vertically into four or six wedges, depending on the size of the pineapple, leaving on the skin and the leaves. Cut the hard core from each wedge. Pipe on a squiggle of meringue (prepared from 2 egg whites and 2 oz caster sugar) and brown in a moderate oven.

Baked Rice   Serves 4

  3 Tbsp round or broken rice
  1 oz margarine
  1 Tbsp sugar
  1 pt soya milk

Spread an ovenware dish with margarine. Add the rice and sugar. Pour in the milk. Bake in a slow oven for 2 hrs.

Rice Pudding   Serves 4

  1 pt soya milk
  sugar to taste
  3 oz round *or* broken rice

Simmer all together until rice is tender.

Rice Imperatrice

Serves 4

1 pt Rice Pudding
4–6 oz mix of chopped cherries, peaches,
    and pineapple
½ pt red table jelly

Prepare Rice Pudding, and allow to cool. Fold in the mixture of chopped cherries, peaches, and pineapple. Turn into a shallow serving-dish. Pour over ½ pt cooled red table jelly. Put aside to set. Pipe with Decorating Cream (p. 40).

Scotch Trifle

Serves 4

Snowcake (p. 152)
2 Tbsp sherry
mixed tinned fruit (4–6 oz approx)
½ pt custard (p. 38)
Decorating Cream (p. 40)
bitter chocolate

Spread the bottom of a 2 pt serving-dish with a generous layer of jam. Cover with a layer of Snowcake cut into fingers. Sprinkle on some chopped tinned fruit (peaches, pears, cherries, etc.) Moisten, but do not soak, with some of the juice of the fruit and/or the sherry. Top with custard made with soya milk. Allow to cool and set. Pipe with Decorating Cream. Sprinkle with grated bitter chocolate.

Semolina Pudding

Serves 4

1 pt soya milk
sugar to taste
2 oz semolina

Boil the milk and sugar. Sprinkle in the semolina, gradually, stirring to avoid lumps. Cook for 10 mins.

Semolina Jam Meringue
Serves 4

> 1 pt Semolina Pudding (p. 141)
> jam for spreading
> 1 white of egg
> ½ lb seedless jam

Prepare Semolina Pudding. Pour into a serving-dish, and allow to cool. Spread with jam.

Beat a white of egg with the ½ lb of jam (using either an electric or rotary whisk) until mixture is stiff enough to "peak". Heap on to the semolina, or pipe on through a meringue tube.

Steamed Jam Roll (Roly-Poly)
Serves 4

> 8 oz self-raising flour
> 2 oz sugar
> 3 oz margarine
> 6 oz (approx.) water
> ½ tsp salt
> jam

Rub the margarine through the flour, salt and sugar. Add enough water to mix to a soft dough. Pin out to about ¼-inch thickness. Spread with jam. Roll up lightly. Wrap in oiled greaseproof paper. Steam for 1½–2 hrs. Serve with Jam Sauce (p. 39) or custard made with soya milk (p. 38).

Steamed Fruit Pudding
Serves 4

> 8 oz self-raising flour
> 3 oz margarine
> 2 oz sugar
> 1 tsp mixed spice
> 2 oz of currants, *or* raisins, *or* sultanas, *or* mixed fruit

Rub the margarine through the flour. Mix in the other ingredients. Add enough soya milk or water to form a stiff batter. Fill into a margarined basin, cover with foil, and steam for about 1½ hrs.

Spotted Dick

Follow recipe above, using currants only without spice.

Sultana Pudding

Follow recipe above, using sultanas only without spice.

College Pudding

Follow recipe above, using mixed fruit with spice.

Sorbets

Orange Sorbet

> ½ pt orange juice
> ½ pt warm water
> 4 oz sugar
> grated zest of 2 oranges
> 2 egg whites

Dissolve the sugar in the warm water. Allow to cool. Mix in the orange juice and zest. Pour into a tray and put into the freezer at its lowest setting. When the mixture becomes slushy, stir well, breaking up any solid parts. Freeze for a further hour, and again mix well. Beat the egg whites stiffly, and fold into the orange mixture. Return to freezer, and freeze till firm.

Apricot Sorbet

Liquidise a 14 oz (400 gram) tin of apricots. Make up with water to 1 pt. Proceed as for Orange Sorbet.

Peach Sorbet

Proceed as for Apricot Sorbet.

Raspberry Sorbet

With tinned raspberries, proceed as for Apricot Sorbet. With fresh raspberries, liquidise 12 oz fresh raspberries with 6 oz caster sugar. Make up with water to 1 pt. Strain, and proceed as for Orange Sorbet.

Blackcurrant Sorbet

Can be produced by suitably diluting a blackcurrant cordial (such as Ribena) and proceeding as for Orange Sorbet.

Baking

Nearly all commercial bakery products contain either butter or eggs, so that we have little choice except to depend on home-produced articles.

Wrapped sliced bread from the supermarket shelf contains neither dairy products nor eggs; and so on that count, is safe enough for the diet. It does, however, contain additives to extend shelf life which are probably best avoided. With home-made bread, on the other hand, there are no such drawbacks; and an advantage is that fibre content can be controlled to suit personal preference.

Bread is simple to make, and there is no need to give a recipe for it here, since white, wheatmeal and wholemeal bread flour are readily available in all food stores and every packet carries a good recipe for a basic loaf. Just remember to use margarine where the recipe calls for lard. Note, also, that there is now on the market a dried yeast which does not require creaming, as it is simply mixed into the flour. I recommend its use.

The recipes which follow are for a few examples of the cakes and buns that can be easily prepared for afternoon tea and are suitable for the diet.

Buckwheat Pancakes (Blinis)   *Makes about 12*

> 3 oz self-raising flour
> 4 oz buckwheat flour
> ½ pt soya milk
> 1 stiffly beaten white of egg
> 1 tsp sugar
> 1 oz melted margarine
> ½ tsp salt

Mix all ingredients, except the egg white, to a smooth batter. Fold in the beaten egg white, and cook as for drop scones on a girdle or in a thick-based frying-pan.

Blinis

These are of Russian origin and are traditionally made there with yeast, as follows.

Cream 1 tsp dried yeast with a little sugar and soya milk. When frothy, mix into the batter made as above, using plain instead of self-raising flour. Leave in a warm place till the batter has doubled its volume. Fold in the beaten egg white, and cook as above.

Coconut Cakes   *Makes about 20*

> 8 oz self-raising flour
> 4 oz margarine
> 4 oz sugar
> 2 oz desiccated coconut
> 2 egg whites

Beat the sugar and margarine to a cream. Beat the egg whites stiffly. Mix into the creamed sugar and margarine, and beat for 3–4 mins. Mix in flour and coconut. Drop in spoonfuls on to an oiled baking tray. Cook in a hot oven for 8–10 mins.

Drop Scones (Scotch Pancakes)   *Makes 10–12*

> 4 oz self-raising flour
> 4 oz soya milk
> pinch of salt
> 1 oz caster sugar
> 1 tsp oil
> 1 white of egg
> (Note that 4 oz is just less than ¼ pint)

Make a thick batter with the flour, sugar, oil, soya milk and salt. Rest the batter for 15 mins. Beat the egg white not too stiffly. Fold into the batter. Drop with a spoon on to an oiled girdle or thick-based frying-pan.

Flapjacks   *Makes about 12*

> 4 oz oatflakes
> 4 oz syrup

2 oz sugar
2 oz margarine

Melt the syrup, sugar, and margarine, and stir in the oatflakes. Press into a shallow tin. Cook in moderate oven for 30 mins. While still hot, cut into fingers, or triangles. Cool, and separate.

Gingerbread

1 lb self-raising flour
6 oz margarine
8 oz sugar
8 oz treacle
½ tsp salt
4 oz mixed dried fruit
1½ cups warm soya milk
2 tsp ground ginger
1 tsp mixed spice

Rub the margarine through the flour. Add the spice, ginger, salt, and mixed fruit. Mix treacle with the warm milk, and stir into the dry ingredients. Mix to a heavy batter. Bake in a shallow tin for 45 mins in a moderate oven.

Ginger Parkins   *Makes 12–16*

4 oz medium oatmeal
4 oz plain flour
2 oz syrup
2 oz sugar
split almonds
2 oz margarine
½ tsp mixed spice
1 tsp ground ginger
1 tsp baking soda

Melt the syrup, sugar, and margarine, and mix in all dry ingredients. Form into balls (they will collapse into flat biscuits.) Top each with a half almond. Bake in a moderate oven for 15 mins.

Mince Pies

Prepare pies with either sweetcrust (p. 150) or puff pastry (p. 148) filling with the mixture given below.

Mincemeat

2 oz margarine
2 oz raisins
2 oz currants
2 oz soft brown sugar
2 tsp mixed spice
2 oz sultanas
2 oz mixed peel
1 finely chopped cooking apple
2 Tbsp lemon juice

Melt the margarine, and mix into all other ingredients. Store for at least a week in a sealed jar, before using.

Oatflake Fingers
Makes about 12–16

6 oz oatflakes
4 oz margarine
2 oz plain flour
2 oz caster sugar

Melt the margarine, and mix with other ingredients. Press into a shallow tin, to about ½-inch thick. Cook in moderate oven for 20–25 mins. Cut into fingers while still hot. Allow to cool in tin.

Pastry

Puff pastry

It is now possible to buy frozen puff pastry made with only vegetable fat, but this is not available in all food stores. Here is a recipe using solid vegetable frying-oil in place of the traditional butter.

8 oz strong bread flour
1 oz soft margarine
¼ pt very cold water
6 oz solid vegetable oil
1 tsp lemon juice
1 tsp salt

Rub the soft margarine through the flour. Add the salt, lemon juice, and cold water, and mix to a stiff dough. Knead till smooth. Rest dough for 15 mins. Work the vegetable oil till it is plastic. Pin out the dough to the shape of a square leaving the centre thicker than the corners. Place vegetable oil in the centre, and sandwich it into the dough by bringing up and folding over the four corners to the centre. You will now have as much paste above the fat as there is below it.

Pin out the dough to a rectangle approximately 15 ins by 5 ins. Fold into three. Turn through ninety degrees, and pin out again to the same shape and size. Fold again into three. Rest the dough for 20 mins. Repeat the rolling out and folding process twice more. Rest the dough for a further 20 mins. Repeat the entire process, including the resting, twice more. This will give the pastry six turns in all, with a rest of 20 mins after each two turns. Rest the dough for at least another 20 mins before use. It is always advisable, also, to rest puff pastry for 20 mins or so after cutting it into whatever shape you require to make before cooking. Otherwise it will shrink and lose shape.

Note: The pastry must be kept cold throughout the whole process. If the working area is warm, wrap the pastry in plastic and store it in the fridge during the 20-minute rest periods. Puff pastry must always be cooked in a hot oven.

Shortcrust pastry

8 oz plain flour
4 oz margarine
1 Tbsp water

Rub the margarine through the flour till the mixture has the consistency of breadcrumbs. Add the water, and mix to a firm dough.

Sweetcrust pastry

>   8 oz plain flour
>   2 oz caster sugar
>   4 oz margarine
>   1 Tbsp water

Rub margarine through flour as for Shortcrust. Add the sugar.
Add the water, and mix to a firm dough.

Note: Short and Sweetcrust pastry should always be cooked in
a cool to moderate oven.

Potato Scones

>   8 oz freshly mashed potatoes
>   ½ oz margarine
>   2 oz plain flour
>   ½ tsp salt

Allow the potatoes to cool slightly. Mix in the margarine and salt.
Mix in the flour. Dust with flour, and pin out very thinly to 8-inch
rounds. Cut in quarters. Cook on both sides on a hot girdle. Cool,
and fry as required, in margarine.

Scones

Girdle Scones

>   1 lb self-raising flour
>   ¾ pt (approx.) soya milk
>   1 tsp salt

Mix the ingredients to a soft dough, handling it as little as
possible. Pin out on a well-floured surface, to ½-inch thickness.
Cut into rounds or triangles. Brown both sides on a not-too-hot
girdle.

Cooked in one piece about 1-inch thick in a hot oven, the above
becomes soda bread.

Oven Scones

> 8 oz self-raising flour
> 2 oz margarine
> 1½ oz caster sugar
> 6 oz (approx.) soya milk

Rub margarine through flour and sugar. Mix in milk to make a soft dough. Handle dough as little and as lightly as possible. Roll out on a well-floured surface to about 1-inch thickness. Cut into rounds. Cook in a hot oven for 10–12 mins.

The scones may be either dusted with flour or glazed with soya milk before cooking.

Oven scones can be varied by adding sultanas or currants to the dough.

Treacle Scones

Treacle scones are made by replacing the sugar with 1 Tbsp of black treacle.

Wholemeal or Bran Scones

> 4 oz strong white flour
> 6 oz wholemeal flour
> 2 tsp baking powder
> 2 tsp sugar
> 1½ oz margarine
> ¼ pt (approx.) soya milk

Thoroughly mix the two kinds of flour, the baking powder, and the sugar. Rub in the margarine, and mix in the milk to make a soft dough. Pin out to ½-inch thickness. Cut into rounds or triangles. Cook in a hot oven for 10–12 mins.

Scotch Shortbread

> 1 lb plain flour
> 8 oz margarine
> 4 oz caster sugar
> pinch of salt

Mix the flour and sugar and salt. Rub in the margarine, then work mixture to a smooth paste. Shape into 2 flat rounds ¾ inch thick.

(The Scots use special wooden moulds.) Place rounds on a lightly-oiled baking tray. Mark the rounds deeply into 6 or 8 triangles. Prick all over with a fork. Cook for 1 hr in a slow oven.

When cooled, shortbread will keep for a long period in an airtight tin.

Snowcake

> 3 oz cornflour
> 5 oz self-raising flour
> 4 oz caster sugar
> 4 oz margarine
> ½ Tbsp lemon juice
> 3 egg whites

Cream the sugar and margarine till mixture is light and fluffy. Beat in the lemon juice. Beat the whites of egg stiffly, and beat into the creamed margarine and sugar. Continue beating at high speed for 4–5 mins. Mix in flour and cornflour. Cook in a moderately hot oven for 25 mins.

The above quantities will be enough for two 7½-in sandwich tins. Use for jam sandwich, or any gâteau.

Vanilla Slice (Gâteau Millefeuilles)

> 8 oz puff pastry (p. 148)
> 3 Tbsp custard powder
> 1 pt soya milk
> jam
> 1 oz (approx.) margarine
> *Water icing*
> 4 oz icing sugar
> 4 tsp water

Make a pint of custard sauce using the soya milk. Allow to cool.

Pin out a piece of puff pastry to fit a jam roll tin. The pastry will be about ¼ inch thick. Prick all over with a fork. Rest pastry for 20 mins. Cook in a hot oven. Cool on a wire. Cut the pastry in half across its length. Split both halves horizontally.

Fill the split halves with cold custard which has had some margarine beaten through. Spread the top of one half with jam, and place the other half over it, so creating layers as follows: pastry, custard, pastry, jam, pastry, custard, pastry. Cover with a tray, and press with a weight, for an hour or so.

To make the water icing, add water *DROP BY DROP TO ICING SUGAR* until it is just spreadable. Some of the water may be replaced (not added to) by lemon juice.

Spread the top of the cake with water icing. When icing is set, cut the cake into fingers or squares with a sharp, thin-bladed knife which has been dipped in hot water.

Kitchen Equipment

Recommendations for kitchen equipment to help arthritis sufferers, such as the replacement of the common type of cooker with separate hob and waist-height oven, could be just too expensive to contemplate. There are available on the market, however, small inexpensive electric ovens that sit on a bench or table-top and simply plug into a wall-socket. Space limitations may also make the installation of easily reached cupboards impractical, but with a little thought the contents can be arranged so that the most used articles are the most accessible.

Gadgets

Gadgets are available to help to turn on switches and taps and these gadgets can be purchased or can easily be made by any handy person. For example: A piece of plastic pipe is cut in castellations at one end to fit over a tap or switch and a handle is fixed at right angles to the other so that the tap or switch can be pushed rather than turned.

If there is no table-top in the kitchen, then a flap can be fixed to a bench top so that one can sit with knees underneath to work comfortably.

Explore the hardware stores for other gadgets that help. There are grips to unscrew jar tops; scissors with a spring, that have only to be squeezed; wall-fixed tin-openers that hold the can; electric plugs with solid ring grips, and many more ingenious inexpensive articles. It is important, however, that the article is strongly constructed. Tinny articles that twist or break are dangerous.

Knives

The most important tool in any kitchen is a knife. It is also the one which is often given least thought. Always buy the best you can afford. Cheap wobbly knives are dangerous and usually don't cut after the first week. I would recommend having four. 1 × 3″ cook's knife, 1 × 8″ cook's knife, 1 carving knife and 1 palette knife. Knives must be kept sharp. The knife should be able to slide easily through whatever is being cut. A blunt knife needs pressure to get through the article and so is difficult to control – it also makes a poor job. Do not use those nasty little wheel sharpeners. They destroy knives. Ask a kindly butcher, or a craftsman such as a joiner, to put an edge on the knife for you.

Kettles

The traditional design requires an awkward turning action of the wrist for pouring while holding the full weight of the kettle. The modern plastic electric jug is so much lighter and the design allows it to be tilted, without lifting, to fill a tea-pot. If the jug is placed on a raised object, then taller utensils, such as coffee-pots, can also be filled without having to lift.

Cooking pans

Try to avoid thin pans. They burn too easily. They also distort and so develop hot spots that make burning even more likely.

Cast-iron pans are thick and distribute heat well but they are just too heavy. If not cared for, they are subject to rust.

Cast aluminium has a thick enough base and diffuses the heat well. It is of course lighter than pans of similar thickness. After a period it pits, but this takes a long time. Overall it is probably the best type for our purpose. Light, spun aluminium pans should be avoided.

Enamelled steel pans look nice when they are new and with a nonstick coating they are easy to clean, but they chip easily if dropped and nothing looks sleazier than a chipped enamelled pan. They are, however, reasonably light.

Stainless steel pans are generally made from light gauge metal to keep down weight. Stainless steel is a poor conductor of heat so the better pans have a copper bottom, but this tends to add weight and cost. Their great advantage is that they are very easily cleaned and they last for ever.

Glass pans. I approached these with caution, but I have had a glass sauce-pan for years and it has stood up well. It is heavy for its size but it distributes the heat well and is still as easy to clean as ever. It is unusual in that it can be transferred straight from the stove to the microwave or vice-versa – very useful when something cooked on the stove, and which burns easily, needs reheating.

Tinned copper pans were, and to some degree still are, the favoured pans of the great kitchens. They can stand up to hard usage and copper distributes the heat better than anything else, but they are very expensive. The main drawback is that the tinning wears off in time. They can be retinned but the job is costly and it could be difficult to find someone to do it.

A chip pan that heats on the top of the stove should on no account be used. If anything goes wrong, anyone with weak hands or wrists just cannot handle it. The thermostatically controlled electric deep-frier is inexpensive; and, as it sits on a table-top, does not have to be moved.

As with the chip pan, an electric frying-pan is so much safer to use. It will do any frying job except perhaps omelettes. It also makes an excellent, easily controlled griddle for scones and scotch pancakes and crumpets. For some reason the electric frying-pan costs a little more than the chip pan, but it is so easy to control that it is money well spent.

A pressure-cooker is not the favourite tool of the *cordon bleu* cook but it does save a lot of time and fuel. Some instruction books suggest that the pressure can be reduced by running cold water over the cooker, but this means lifting and carrying the cooker to the sink, and should on no account be attempted. Just turn off the heat and allow the pressure to subside. Most models require the lid to be turned to lock or release, and this, too, could prove to be difficult.

Liquidiser or blender

These are so cheap that it is folly to be without one. A liquidiser can reduce any soup to a smooth cream in seconds. It will make bread crumbs from fresh bread; grind down soya beans for soya milk; reduce garlic or fresh ginger to paste and do many similar tasks that would otherwise require hard work and strong wrists. It is a must.

Food mixers

Of the food mixers there are various bench models on the market, but those in the cheaper range are limited in their uses. The more expensive models have a planetary movement, and with their many attachments for grinding, slicing and mincing are very fine tools indeed. There are also some very useful hand-held electric mixers available. The rechargeable battery type is especially useful, because it can be carried all round the kitchen and is completely safe. It is highly recommended.

Food processor

In the average home the food processor is rarely used to anything like its full potential.

The food processor can slice pounds of vegetables in seconds. It can convert large quantities of raw meat into sausage meat quickly and without effort. The snag is that most households do not cater for larger numbers. Mostly the quantities they use are measured in ounces rather than pounds and a sharp knife can do the job faster than the food processor can be set up. When the job is finished the knife is wiped clean in seconds. The food processor has to be dismantled, and the various parts cleaned separately, then stored on the special rack.

At the more expensive end of the market there are models with attachments that mince and grind and are powerful enough to mix a 3 lb bread dough. These are well worth considering.

Microwave oven

This piece of equipment, like the food processor, is generally under-utilised. It is used mostly to defrost and to heat up television meals and such like. A lot of cooking can be done on it, but very rarely is after the initial novelty has worn off. The newer, more sophisticated, and much more expensive models can turn out food that compares in appearance with traditional methods, but the inexpensive models cannot. The instruction manual and the enthusiasts can explain how the snags can be overcome, but the average user just cannot be bothered. The lower priced models are low powered, and, although they can cook one baked potato in about 6 minutes it takes another 6 minutes for each and every other potato. The conventional oven cooks a number of potatoes in little more time than the microwave and the end product is better. *The great advantage of a microwave for the arthritis sufferer is that, with the proper dishes, the food can be heated while the dishes themselves remain cool. This makes handling so much safer.*

Metric Conversion Tables

Weights		Liquid Measures	
Imperial	**Metric** *(to nearest 25g)*	**Imperial**	**Metric**
¼ oz	7 g	1 fl oz	25 ml
½ oz	15 g	2 fl oz	50 ml
1 oz	25 g	3 fl oz	75 ml
2 oz	50 g	4 fl oz	100 ml
3 oz	75 g	5 fl oz / ¼ pt	150 ml
4 oz / ¼ lb	100 g	6 fl oz	175 ml
5 oz	150 g	⅓ pt	190 ml
6 oz	175 g	7 fl oz	200 ml
7 oz	200 g	8 fl oz	225 ml
8 oz / ½ lb	225 g	9 fl oz	250 ml
9 oz	250 g	10 fl oz / ½ pt	275 ml
10 oz	275 g	11 fl oz	300 ml
11 oz	300 g	12 fl oz	350 ml
12 oz / ¾ lb	350 g	13 fl oz	375 ml
13 oz	375 g	⅔ pt	380 ml
14 oz	400 g	14 fl oz	400 ml
15 oz	425 g	15 fl oz / ¾ pt	425 ml
16 oz / 1 lb	450 g	20 fl oz / 1 pt	570 ml
1½ lb	675 g	1½ pt	850 ml
2 lb	900 g	2 pt	1.15 l

Oven Temperature Chart

VERY HOT	475–500°F	240–250°C
HOT	425–450°F	220–230°C
MODERATELY HOT	375–400°F	190–200°C
MODERATE	350°F	180°C
MODERATELY SLOW	325°F	170°C
SLOW	300°F	150°C
VERY SLOW	250°F	130°C

Index